Common Childhood Illnesses - Epidemiology, Diagnosis, and Treatment

Edited by Öner Özdemir

Published in London, United Kingdom

Common Childhood Illnesses - Epidemiology, Diagnosis, and Treatment
http://dx.doi.org/10.5772/intechopen.1008603
Edited by Öner Özdemir

Contributors
Ann Brai, Derryl Joseph Miller, Ebenovbe Idemudia, Festus Mulakoli, Hadia R. Mruma, Hippolite O. Amadi, Kubra Yırgın, Mehmet Halil Celiksoy, Sofia A. Giannini, Sumayya S. Mussa, Taylor N. Parrish, Trisha Lea Miller

First published in London, United Kingdom, 2026 by IntechOpen
IntechOpen is the global imprint of INTECHOPEN LIMITED, registered in England and Wales, registration number: 11086078, 167-169 Great Portland Street, London, W1W 5PF, United Kingdom

For EU product safety concerns: IN TECH d.o.o., Prolaz Marije Krucifikse Kozulić 3, 51000 Rijeka, Croatia, info@intechopen.com or visit our website at intechopen.com.

British Library Cataloguing-in-Publication Data
A catalogue record for this book is available from the British Library

Common Childhood Illnesses - Epidemiology, Diagnosis, and Treatment
Edited by Öner Özdemir
p. cm.
Print ISBN 978-1-83634-347-9
Online ISBN 978-1-83634-346-2
eBook (PDF) ISBN 978-1-83634-348-6

Meet the editor

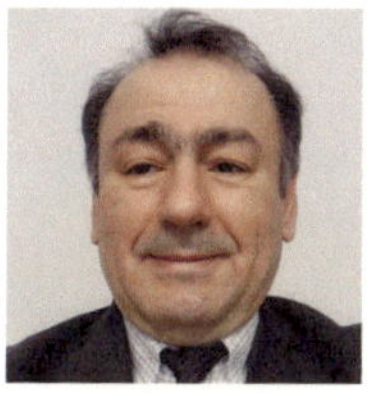

Prof. Dr. Öner Özdemir was born in Alaplı, Zonguldak, Türkiye, in 1965. He graduated from the İstanbul Medical School at İstanbul University and became a medical doctor in 1989. Dr. Özdemir did his pediatric residency at the Department of Pediatrics in the Children's Hospital, İstanbul Medical School, İstanbul, Türkiye. His clinical fellowship training was completed at the Pediatric Allergy/Immunology division of Louisiana State University Health Sciences Center, New Orleans, LA. Dr. Özdemir's research areas include: LAK-cell generation and cell-mediated cytotoxicity, human mast cell development and mast cell-mediated cytotoxicity, and apoptosis-related research. Dr. Özdemir's clinical research areas are mastocytosis, hereditary angioedema, and chronic urticaria. Dr. Özdemir has authored over 400 international and national publications, as well as more than 20 chapters, spanning various research areas.

Contents

Preface

This book, *Common Childhood Illnesses - Epidemiology, Diagnosis, and Treatment,* focuses on common childhood diseases, ranging from infections to allergic diseases, in 5 chapters divided into 4 sections.

The chapter in section 1 reviews malnutrition during childhood. Although it remains rare, childhood malnutrition can still occur in environments with limited resources. This first section will discuss developments and innovations in the epidemiology, diagnosis, and treatment of malnutrition.

Chapter 1 in Section 2 discusses global trends in neonatal sepsis. A Scopus bibliometric analysis of publications on neonatal sepsis over the past 10 years (2015-2025) is conducted to examine global trends in this field.

Chapter 2 in Section 2 discusses neonatal survival against LMIC odds. A case study of ten newborns in critical condition who were saved by a new initiative is being discussed, and the benefits of this approach are being explored. This interesting section would be particularly beneficial for neonatologists to review.

Chapter 1 in Section 3 discusses the treatment of drug-resistant epilepsy. Treatment-resistant epilepsy is one of the most complex issues in neurology. Sometimes, surgery can provide a definitive solution to this problem. This section explains the stages of preoperative evaluation for definitive treatment.

The chapter in Section 4 discusses allergic rhinitis. Allergic rhinitis and asthma are the most common respiratory diseases in children. As with all allergic diseases, the incidence of this disease has increased in recent years. Although its diagnosis and treatment are less complex than in adults, its increasing incidence makes it particularly problematic, especially around adolescence. Our colleagues, who are experts in the field, have covered this section in considerable detail.

In conclusion, I hope it proves helpful to our readers, and I look forward to meeting you in many more upcoming books.

I want to thank our Publishing Process Managers, Mateo Belir, Senior Commissioning Editor, Iva Simcic Mance, and the editorial team.

I want to express my gratitude to my dear wife, Seval Hülya Özdemir, and my dear daughter, Berrin Nikame Özdemir, for their moral support during the preparation of this book.

Öner Özdemir
Sakarya Research and Training Hospital,
Division of Pediatric Allergy and Immunology,
Sakarya University Medical Faculty,
Sakarya, Türkiye

Section 1

Childhood Malnutrition

Chapter 1

Childhood Malnutrition: Epidemiology, Diagnosis, and Treatment in Low-Resource Settings

Sumayya S. Mussa and Hadia R. Mruma

Abstract

Childhood malnutrition remains one of the most critical global health challenges, disproportionately affecting children in low-resource and conflict-affected settings, where it significantly contributes to child morbidity, mortality, and developmental delays. This chapter provides a comprehensive overview of the epidemiology, diagnosis, treatment, and policy landscape of childhood malnutrition, with a focus on resource-limited, including conflict-affected, settings. Globally, over 148 million children are stunted, and 45 million are wasted, with Sub-Saharan Africa and parts of Asia bearing the heaviest burden. Factors such as poverty and maternal education are compounded by conflict and displacement, creating persistent barriers to child nutrition. The diagnosis of malnutrition in low-resource environments relies heavily on anthropometric tools such as MUAC and WHZ, as well as clinical signs like bilateral edema. Field challenges, ranging from tool shortages to limited trained personnel, are increasingly addressed through community health worker training and digital innovations. Treatment strategies emphasize both community-based management (CMAM) and facility-based care, incorporating the use of ready-to-use therapeutic foods (RUTF), micronutrient supplementation, and adherence to World Health Organization's (WHO's) ten-step treatment protocol. Broader nutrition-sensitive interventions, such as WASH (water, sanitation, and hygiene) improvements, food security programs, and health system integration, are essential to preventing relapse and sustaining recovery. Monitoring and evaluation remain central to program effectiveness, especially in unstable or fragile settings. The chapter concludes with policy recommendations emphasizing the need for multisectoral coordination, data-driven decision-making, and strong political commitment. Through integrated, evidence-based approaches, significant strides can be made in reducing the burden of childhood malnutrition and ensuring every child's right to health and development.

Keywords: childhood malnutrition, low-resource settings, nutrition assessment, conflict zones, under nutrition, disease of poverty

1. Introduction

1.1 Definition and forms of childhood malnutrition

Childhood malnutrition remains one of the most pressing global public health challenges of the twenty-first century. Despite decades of progress in child health and survival, malnutrition continues to contribute to nearly half of all deaths among children under 5 years of age, particularly in low- and middle-income countries [1]. The term "malnutrition" encompasses a broad spectrum of conditions resulting from deficiencies, excesses, or imbalances in energy and nutrient intake. Among children, the most prevalent forms include stunting (low height-for-age), wasting (low weight-for-height), underweight (low weight-for-age), and various micronutrient deficiencies that impair immunity, growth, and cognitive development [2].

The burden of childhood malnutrition is unevenly distributed across the globe, with Sub-Saharan Africa (SSA) and South Asia disproportionately affected. However, the impact of conflict, political instability, natural disasters, and displacement has also contributed to rising levels of malnutrition in other regions, including parts of the Middle East, North Africa, and Central America [3]. In conflict settings such as Syria, Sudan, Somalia, and Gaza, malnutrition rates have reached emergency thresholds as food systems collapse and healthcare infrastructure becomes severely disrupted [4]. These settings pose unique challenges to prevention and treatment, with limited access to essential services and high rates of population displacement.

This chapter provides a comprehensive overview of the epidemiology, diagnosis, and treatment of childhood malnutrition in low-resource and conflict-affected settings. It explores the global magnitude of the problem, identifies vulnerable populations, and outlines practical approaches to diagnosis and case management. By highlighting current evidence and programmatic experiences, especially from humanitarian emergencies, the chapter aims to equip health professionals, policymakers, and development partners with the knowledge and tools to respond effectively to childhood malnutrition, ultimately contributing to the achievement of the sustainable development goals (SDGs).

1.2 Impact on child survival and development

The consequences of malnutrition are profound and far-reaching, particularly in the early years of life when growth and development are most critical. Malnutrition contributes to nearly 45% of all deaths among children under 5 years of age, translating to over three million preventable deaths annually[5]. Undernourished children have a weakened immune response, making them significantly more susceptible to common childhood infections such as pneumonia, diarrhea, malaria, and tuberculosis. These infections, in turn, worsen nutritional status, creating a vicious cycle of illness and undernutrition[6].

Moreover, micronutrient deficiencies further exacerbate health risks. Deficiencies in vitamin A impair immune function and vision, iron deficiency leads to anemia and poor cognitive development, and inadequate iodine intake hinders neurodevelopment and growth [7]. Children who survive early malnutrition often face long-term physical and mental impairments [8]. Stunted children are less likely to perform well in school, have reduced educational attainment, and often experience lower earning potential and economic productivity in adulthood. In addition, the adverse effects of childhood undernutrition can extend across generations. Malnourished girls are more likely to grow into undernourished women and give birth to low-birth-weight infants, perpetuating the cycle of poverty, poor health, and underdevelopment [9].

1.3 Relevance to global goals

Tackling childhood malnutrition is essential for achieving global development targets, particularly those outlined in the SDGs [10]. SDG 2 aims to end hunger and all forms of malnutrition by 2030, while SDG 3 focuses on ensuring healthy lives and promoting well-being for all. Addressing childhood malnutrition aligns directly with SDG 2.2, which calls for the elimination of all forms of malnutrition, including stunting and wasting; and SDG 3.2, which targets a reduction in under-five mortality to at least 25 per 1,000 live births [11].

Nutrition also intersects with many other development goals, including those related to education, gender equality, economic growth, and climate action. Achieving the global nutrition targets will require comprehensive, multisectoral strategies that go beyond the health sector. These include scaling up evidence-based interventions such as exclusive breastfeeding, appropriate complementary feeding, vitamin and mineral supplementation, treatment of acute malnutrition, and promotion of food security [12]. Strengthening health systems, improving water and sanitation, enhancing maternal education, and ensuring access to nutritious foods are all critical components of this effort. In addition, investment in nutrition yields high economic returns. Ultimately, addressing malnutrition is not only a moral and health imperative; it is a strategic development priority.

2. Global epidemiology of childhood malnutrition

2.1 Global context and magnitude

Childhood malnutrition remains a widespread public health challenge, particularly in low-resource and humanitarian settings. According to the 2023 UNICEF- World Health Organization (WHO)-World Bank Joint Malnutrition Estimates, approximately 148 million children under the age of five are stunted, 45 million are wasted, and nearly half a billion suffer from one or more forms of micronutrient deficiency. These alarming figures underscore the magnitude of the problem and its persistence, despite global efforts to improve child nutrition. The distribution of malnutrition is not uniform; the greatest burden is carried by SSA and South Asia, where poverty, food insecurity, poor health systems, and inadequate maternal nutrition exacerbate the crisis [2]. In South Asia, for instance, over 34% of children are stunted, with India alone accounting for nearly one-third of the global burden of stunting [13].

The situation is further compounded by conflict and climate-related crises. In countries with ongoing wars, political instability, and natural disasters, food systems have been severely disrupted, populations displaced, and health and sanitation infrastructure has collapsed [14]. Malnutrition levels in these areas have crossed emergency thresholds, often exceeding 15% global acute malnutrition (GAM) rates, as defined by the WHO [4]. In Somalia, over 1.5 million children are projected to suffer from acute malnutrition due to the compounding effects of prolonged drought and insecurity [15]. Similarly, the civil conflict in Sudan displaced over six million people in 2023, severely interrupting nutrition and health services for more than three million acutely malnourished children [16]. In the Gaza Strip, repeated cycles of violence and restricted humanitarian access have left thousands of children at risk of severe nutritional deficiencies due to the destruction of food stores, blockade-induced shortages, and limited access to clean water [17].

2.2 Regional distribution and hotspots

The burden of malnutrition is not evenly distributed, with certain regions facing alarmingly high prevalence. SSA records some of the most severe malnutrition indicators globally. In many SSA countries, stunting rates exceed 30%, and in some cases rise above 40%. Wasting rates in emergency-prone or food-insecure regions typically range between 5% and 10%, but can exceed 15% during humanitarian crises. Contributing factors include chronic food insecurity, recurrent infections, limited maternal healthcare, and inadequate access to essential nutrition and sanitation services[18]. For instance, Nigeria reports a national stunting rate of 37% and a wasting rate of 7% among children under five, according to the 2022 Nigeria Demographic and Health Survey (NDHS) [19]. In Ethiopia, the 2023 Demographic and Health Survey found 37% of children stunted and 7% wasted [20]. In countries facing protracted conflict, such as South Sudan and Somalia, acute malnutrition levels often cross WHO-defined emergency thresholds[14]. In 2023, Somalia's national wasting prevalence reached 16%, particularly in regions impacted by drought and displacement [21].

Tanzania continues to face a significant burden of childhood malnutrition despite relative political stability and improvements in health sector investments. According to the 2022–2023 Tanzania Demographic and Health Survey (TDHS), 30% of children under five are stunted, with higher rates observed in rural regions such as Rukwa, Kigoma, and Songwe. Wasting stands at 3.5%, while underweight prevalence is approximately 12%. Key contributing factors include poor maternal nutrition, limited access to diverse foods, early weaning practices, and low household income [22]. National programs such as the National Multi-Sectoral Nutrition Action Plan (NMNAP) have been implemented, but persistent inequalities in access to health and nutrition services remain a barrier.

The Democratic Republic of Congo (DRC) presents one of the most severe and complex nutrition crises on the continent, exacerbated by decades of armed conflict, political instability, and displacement. In 2023, an estimated 42% of children under five were stunted and 6% were wasted, with some conflict-affected eastern provinces, such as Ituri, North Kivu, and South Kivu, reporting even higher rates [23]. Food insecurity affects over 25 million people in the country, and recurring outbreaks of infectious diseases, such as measles, cholera, and malaria, have further strained the health system. Access to essential services is frequently hindered by insecurity, infrastructure breakdown, and displacement, making it difficult to deliver sustained nutrition interventions.

South Asia continues to bear a disproportionate burden of child undernutrition. The region has the highest global prevalence of wasting, at 14.8%, and a stunting prevalence of approximately 31.7% [18]. India alone contributes nearly 40 million stunted children to the global total. Key drivers in this region include poor maternal nutrition, high rates of adolescent pregnancies, inadequate sanitation, and suboptimal infant feeding practices. Despite economic growth and expanded health infrastructure, persistent inequalities and cultural practices hinder widespread improvements in child nutrition.

In the Middle East and North Africa (MENA), malnutrition is increasingly driven by conflict and displacement. Prolonged emergencies in countries such as Syria, Yemen, and Sudan have devastated food systems, healthcare infrastructure, and access to clean water [24]. In Yemen alone, over 2.2 million children under five were acutely malnourished in 2023, with approximately 540,000 children experiencing severe acute malnutrition (SAM) requiring life-saving treatment [25]. In Syria and Sudan, the combination of insecurity, limited humanitarian access, and a collapsing health system has led to rising rates of both wasting and stunting.

2.3 Conflict-affected regions

Armed conflict is one of the most potent amplifiers of child malnutrition, as it disrupts food availability, displaces populations, damages health infrastructure, and restricts humanitarian operations. In Syria, years of civil war have eroded the healthcare system and water, sanitation, and hygiene (WASH) services, leading to poor hygiene, food scarcity, and reduced access to immunization and nutrition interventions [26]. In Sudan, renewed conflict in regions such as Darfur and Blue Nile has displaced millions and severely disrupted nutrition services in internally displaced persons (IDP) camps. Humanitarian access remains limited due to insecurity and bureaucratic obstacles, placing children at heightened risk of acute malnutrition and mortality [27].

Similarly, Somalia has faced successive droughts, political instability, and insecurity, resulting in repeated nutrition emergencies. In 2023, the Food Security and Nutrition Analysis Unit (FSNAU) reported national wasting rates exceeding 16% in several regions, particularly among displaced populations and pastoralist communities affected by failed rains and livestock losses [15]. In all these contexts, humanitarian responses are often delayed or inadequate, and children's nutritional status deteriorates rapidly due to a lack of access to food, clean water, healthcare, and safe shelter.

2.4 Special populations: Refugees and internally displaced children

Among the most vulnerable populations to the effects of malnutrition are forcibly displaced children, including refugees, asylum seekers, and IDP. In 2023, the United Nations High Commissioner for Refugees (UNHCR) estimated that more than 43 million children were forcibly displaced worldwide due to conflict, persecution, or climate-related disasters [28]. In refugee and IDP camps, food insecurity is often exacerbated by poor dietary diversity, limited maternal care, and unsafe water supplies. Health services in camp settings are frequently overwhelmed, and children face increased risks of disease and undernutrition. Studies have shown that the prevalence of acute malnutrition in refugee children can be two to three times higher than in surrounding host communities [28]. Despite global humanitarian efforts, gaps in funding, insecurity, and policy constraints continue to hinder the delivery of timely and comprehensive nutrition interventions in displacement settings.

3. Determinants of malnutrition

3.1 Immediate, underlying, and basic causes

Childhood malnutrition results from a complex interplay of factors that can be categorized into immediate, underlying, and basic causes, as described in the UNICEF conceptual framework. Immediate causes include inadequate dietary intake and frequent infections such as diarrhea, pneumonia, and parasitic diseases, which increase nutrient loss or hinder absorption. Underlying causes involve food insecurity at the household level, inadequate care practices, poor sanitation, and limited access to quality healthcare. At a deeper level, basic causes encompass broader systemic issues such as poverty, weak governance, inequality, and limited education, especially for women and girls. These structural issues affect the availability of and access to essential services and resources required for adequate nutrition [1–2].

3.2 How conflict, poverty, and climate interact

In fragile settings, conflict, poverty, and climate change often interact to create chronic nutrition emergencies. Armed conflict disrupts food production, destroys infrastructure, and displaces populations, reducing access to food, healthcare, and clean water. Countries such as Sudan, Yemen, and Syria have experienced long-standing conflicts that have severely impacted food systems and child health. Poverty further exacerbates malnutrition by limiting a household's ability to access diverse and nutritious food or afford healthcare. Climate change introduces environmental shocks such as prolonged droughts, flooding, and erratic rainfall, all of which affect agricultural productivity. The convergence of these three factors in regions such as the Sahel and the Horn of Africa has resulted in recurrent food insecurity and elevated rates of SAM [3–5].

3.3 Gender and maternal education

Gender inequality and maternal education significantly influence childhood nutrition outcomes. Educated mothers are more likely to practice exclusive breastfeeding, seek appropriate healthcare, and adopt hygienic practices. Even primary education has been associated with improved child survival and nutritional status. Conversely, women with limited education and decision-making power often struggle to access and allocate resources for proper childcare. Early and repeated pregnancies also increase the risk of maternal undernutrition and low birth weight infants. In many resource-limited settings, systemic gender discrimination restricts women's access to education, healthcare, and income, thereby perpetuating a cycle of malnutrition across generations [29].

4. Diagnosis, challenges, and innovation in resource-limited and emergency settings

4.1 Clinical examination and anthropometric tools in diagnosis

In low-resource and emergency settings, the diagnosis of malnutrition in children relies primarily on clinical examination and anthropometric tools due to the limited availability of laboratory diagnostics. These frontline approaches are cost-effective, simple to use, and suitable for both facility-based and community-level assessments.

Clinical examination is crucial for identifying signs of SAM that may not be immediately evident through measurements alone. The most important clinical sign is bilateral pitting edema, which is a hallmark of Kwashiorkor. This is assessed by gently pressing on the tops of both feet for a few seconds; if a pit remains after lifting the fingers, the child is considered to have nutritional edema and is classified as having SAM regardless of other indicators. Other clinical signs, such as visible wasting, lethargy, skin changes, or hair discoloration, can support the diagnosis but are less specific and often subjective.

Anthropometric measurements are standardized tools that provide objective criteria to assess the severity of malnutrition [30]. The most commonly used measurement is the mid–upper arm circumference (MUAC). It is preferred in community and emergency settings due to its simplicity and the fact that it does not require weighing scales or height boards. An MUAC of less than 11.5 cm indicates SAM, while a measurement between 11.5 and 12.5 cm reflects moderate acute malnutrition (MAM). Weight-for-Height Z-score (WHZ) is another key method, used mainly in health facilities. A WHZ below -3 standard deviations from the median is diagnostic of SAM, and a score between -3 and -2 indicates MAM. While WHZ offers a more detailed nutritional profile, it requires functional scales and height boards, which may be unavailable in some contexts.

Because access to laboratory tests (e.g. serum albumin, electrolytes, or micronutrient levels) is rare in humanitarian and rural settings, clinical and anthropometric approaches remain the cornerstone of malnutrition diagnosis. These methods allow rapid triage and decision-making and are endorsed by the WHO and UNICEF for use in Integrated Management of Acute Malnutrition (IMAM) programs.

4.2 Challenges in diagnosis

Field diagnosis of malnutrition in humanitarian emergencies is fraught with logistical and operational challenges. Equipment such as weighing scales and height boards may be unavailable or unreliable. Health workers are often overburdened and may not receive adequate training. Insecurity or poor road conditions can restrict access to affected populations[31]. Cultural beliefs and stigma may prevent caregivers from participating in screening. In some settings, caregivers may fear that malnourished children will be taken away or blamed for poor care, discouraging their participation in treatment programs. These challenges can delay the identification and management of malnourished children, increasing the risk of complications or death [32].

4.3 Screening innovations: Digital tools and rapid kits

To address these barriers, innovative approaches have emerged. Mobile health (mHealth) tools, such as smartphone-based MUAC apps and image-based diagnosis software, are being introduced in parts of SSA to support community health workers [33]. These tools aim to improve accuracy and coverage while reducing the need for specialized equipment. Digital innovations also support community-led models like Community MUAC (C-MUAC), where mothers are trained to measure their children's arms at home. Studies in Africa have shown this approach to be effective in detecting malnutrition early [34]. In addition, point-of-care diagnostics and rapid test kits for micronutrient deficiencies, such as vitamin A and iron, are in development, though they are not yet widely adopted due to cost and infrastructure needs [35].

5. Treatment and intervention strategies for childhood malnutrition

Effective treatment of childhood malnutrition in low-resource and emergency settings requires a dual approach: direct nutrition-specific interventions to treat acute conditions, and broader system-level actions to address underlying drivers. Addressing it requires a comprehensive approach that combines clinical treatment with broad-based intervention strategies aimed at both immediate recovery and long-term prevention. The WHO and UNICEF provide robust guidelines that shape both community-based and facility-based care, including therapeutic feeding, medical management, micronutrient support, and follow-up. When properly implemented, these interventions significantly reduce child mortality and long-term disability.

5.1 Community-based management of acute malnutrition (CMAM)

The CMAM model, developed in response to limitations in facility access, allows the treatment of uncomplicated SAM at the community level, enabling early identification and decentralized treatment of uncomplicated SAM and MAM in the community without requiring hospitalization. It is built on the premise that most children with acute malnutrition can be treated at home with ready-to-use therapeutic foods (RUTF), provided they have no medical complications and can eat orally. This model improves early detection, coverage, and cost-effectiveness, especially in rural and conflict-affected regions. Community health workers and caregivers are trained to identify malnutrition using MUAC tapes and simple clinical signs, referring complicated cases to health facilities. Community health workers play a vital role in active case finding, nutritional screening, and follow-up. This decentralized approach has proven effective in improving access and coverage, particularly in rural or conflict-affected regions[6].

CMAM: This model is especially vital in rural, conflict-affected, and nomadic populations where access to hospitals is limited.

5.2 Key components of CMAM:

- **Outpatient therapeutic program (OTP):** Children with SAM, aged 6–59 months, who have a good appetite and no medical complications are treated at home with **RUTF,** such as Plumpy'Nut. Follow-up visits occur weekly or biweekly to monitor MUAC, weight gain, and clinical signs. Routine **vitamin A** supplementation and deworming are provided.

- **Supplementary feeding program (SFP):** For children with MAM MUAC 11.5–12.5 cm or WHZ -2 to -3 standard deviations (SD), **Ready-to-Use Supplementary Foods (RUSF)** or fortified blended flours, such as **Super Cereal Plus,** are provided in community settings.

- **Community mobilization and screening:** Community health workers and volunteers play a critical role in early detection by using **MUAC tapes**, conducting active case finding, and referring children who require inpatient care.

CMAM has increased coverage and decreased mortality globally, with cure rates exceeding 75% in well-functioning programs.[36]

5.3 Facility-based treatment

Facility-based management is essential for children with SAM who present with complications such as hypoglycemia, hypothermia, infections, or shock. The WHO outlines a structured "10-step approach," which is critical in the management of patients with SAM to stabilize them before transitioning to rehabilitation and discharge. This approach includes treating and preventing hypoglycemia and hypothermia, correcting dehydration carefully, treating infections empirically, correcting micronutrient deficiencies, and initiating cautious feeding followed by catch-up growth and emotional support[30]. These children are at high risk of death and must be treated in stabilization centers or hospitals with trained staff and essential supplies.

Health facilities, especially district hospitals and referral centers, also offer therapeutic feeding with formulae such as F-75 and F-100 and provide monitoring for comorbidities, anemia, or tuberculosis. However, in many low-resource settings, limitations such as inadequate staffing, poor infrastructure, and lack of equipment pose significant challenges to optimal care delivery.

5.4 Admission criteria:

MUAC <11.5 cm or WHZ <-3 SD **with** any of the following:

- Bilateral pedal edema

- Poor appetite (failed appetite test with RUTF)

- Medical complications (e.g. hypothermia, shock, pneumonia, sepsis).

5.5 WHO ten-step protocol for inpatient management

The WHO outlines a standardized **ten-step approach** for the **inpatient treatment of children with SAM** who present with complications [30]. These children are at high risk of death and require careful clinical and nutritional management. The steps begin with emergency stabilization and proceed to nutritional rehabilitation and follow-up, the key steps are summarizes in **Tables 1** and **2**. This structured approach is particularly critical in resource-limited hospitals, where health workers may not be specialized in nutrition or pediatrics.

(1) **Treat/prevent hypoglycemia**: Children with SAM are prone to low blood sugar due to poor feeding and infection. Hypoglycemia must be addressed immediately with 10% glucose or sugary water administered orally or via a nasogastric (NG) tube, and feeding must begin within 30 minutes of admission.

(2) **Treat/prevent hypothermia**: Hypothermia is common and can be fatal in malnourished children. Passive warming, skin-to-skin contact, warm fluids, and maintaining a warm environment are essential.

(3) **Treat/prevent dehydration**: Dehydration signs are unreliable in cases of SAM. ReSoMal (Rehydration Solution for Malnutrition) is administered orally or via an NG tube; intravenous (IV) fluids are given **only** in cases of shock, and with caution.

(4) **Correct electrolyte imbalance**: All children with SAM have hidden deficiencies in potassium and magnesium, as well as excess sodium. These imbalances are corrected by feeding therapeutic milks (F-75/F-100) and avoiding sodium-rich IV fluids.

(5) **Treat infections empirically**: SAM suppresses typical signs of infection, so all children should be treated empirically with broad-spectrum antibiotics (ampicillin + gentamicin).

(6) **Correct micronutrient deficiencies**: Vitamin A is administered upon admission. Iron is withheld during the stabilization phase (due to the risk of increasing infection) and introduced later. Other essential micronutrients, such as zinc, copper, and folate, are included in therapeutic feeds.

(7) **Initiate cautious feeding**: Stabilization begins with F-75, a low-protein, low-energy therapeutic milk designed to prevent refeeding syndrome. Small, frequent feeds are administered using a cup or an NG tube.

(8) **Achieve catch-up growth**: After appetite returns and the clinical condition stabilizes, F-100 or RUTF is introduced to promote rapid weight gain (10–15 g/kg/day).

(9) **Provide sensory stimulation and emotional support**: Psychosocial stimulation, play, and caregiver interaction support cognitive development and recovery.

(10) **Prepare for discharge and follow-up**: Children are discharged based on anthropometric recovery and medical stability. A clear plan for follow-up, continued feeding, and linkage to community support is necessary to prevent relapse.

This approach has been shown to reduce case fatality rates in SAM. In many low-resource settings, however, poor adherence to the protocol due to overcrowded wards, lack of training, or shortages of F-75/F-100 remains a challenge [29–31].

Step	Action	Goal
1	Treat/prevent hypoglycemia	Stabilize blood glucose, prevent seizures/coma
2	Treat/prevent hypothermia	Maintain normal body temperature
3	Treat/prevent dehydration	Rehydrate safely using ReSoMal; avoid fluid overload
4	Correct electrolyte imbalance	Normalize potassium and magnesium; reduce sodium load
5	Treat infections empirically	Address underlying infections and prevent sepsis-related mortality
6	Correct micronutrient deficiencies	Restore essential vitamins and minerals to support immunity and growth
7	Initiate cautious feeding	Avoid refeeding syndrome and promote gradual intake to allow metabolic recovery
8	Achieve catch-up growth	Accelerate weight gain and recovery
9	Provide sensory stimulation and emotional support	Aid mental recovery and parent–child bonding
10	Prepare for discharge and ensure follow-up	Prevent relapse and ensure long-term recovery

Table 1.
WHO's ten steps for the inpatient management of severe acute malnutrition and their goals.

5.6 Feeding protocols in different phases

Phase	Type of feed	Description
Stabilization	F-75	75 kcal/100 mL, low sodium/protein; administered every two to three hours
Transition	F-100 or RUTF	Increased energy (100 kcal/100 mL) for children who are regaining their appetite
Rehabilitation	F-100 or RUTF	High-calorie diets promote catch-up growth (200 kcal/kg/day)
Outpatient care	RUTF (e.g. Plumpy'Nut)	Ready-to-use paste, administered at home with weekly monitoring

Table 2.
Showing feeding protocols in different management strategies for malnutrition.

5.7 Micronutrient and medical management

- **Vitamin A**: Given on Day 1 unless it has already been given within the past month.
- **Antibiotics**: Broad-spectrum (ampicillin and gentamicin) for all children with SAM.
- **Zinc and folate**: Routinely included in feeds or given orally.
- **Iron**: Introduced during the rehabilitation phase once the risk of infection subsides.

- **Deworming**: Albendazole or mebendazole for children over 12 months.

These measures restore immune function, reduce infections, and support metabolic recovery.

6. Monitoring, discharge, and follow-up

Daily monitoring in the inpatient setting includes:

- Temperature, pulse, respiration
- Weight and MUAC
- Edema status
- Appetite

Discharge criteria (from inpatient to outpatient or from OTP to cure):

- MUAC ≥ 12.5 cm or WHZ >–2 SD
- No edema for ≥2 weeks
- Appetite restored
- Completion of antibiotic course
- Adequate weight gain (≥15% of baseline)

Children discharged from inpatient care are transferred to outpatient care (OTP) to complete their nutritional recovery. Regular follow-ups ensure the early detection of relapses.

6.1 Role of caregiver and psychosocial support

Psychosocial support and caregiver involvement are essential to recovery [37]. SAM is associated with developmental delays, poor feeding interactions, and emotional distress. The WHO recommends structured play therapy, caregiver education, and mental health support for long-term cognitive development. Emotional care improves feeding behavior and reduces the risk of relapse [38].

6.2 RUTF and therapeutic feeding

RUTFs are specially formulated, high-energy, nutrient-dense pastes that contain the complete set of nutrients required, often 200 kcal/kg/day, for SAM cases. Typically made from peanuts, milk powder, oil, sugar, and a fortified vitamin–mineral mix, RUTFs are safe for use at home, do not require refrigeration, and have a long shelf life. This makes them ideal for decentralized care in areas without stable electricity or water supplies. RUTFs have been shown to reduce mortality and speed up recovery in children with SAM when used in CMAM programs.

In facility settings, therapeutic feeding begins with F-75 (100 kcal/kg/day), a low-protein, low-sodium milk-based formula given during the stabilization phase when the child's metabolism is compromised. Once stabilized, children transition to F-100, a higher-energy formula used during the rehabilitation phase to promote catch-up growth [30]. For MAM, RUSF are also deployed to treat MAM, often using fortified blended foods such as Super Cereal Plus. The success of therapeutic feeding depends not only on product availability but also on the training of caregivers, cultural acceptability, and consistent supply chains. Programs should be adapted to the context, for example, integrating local foods or using community kitchens during emergencies.

6.3 Micronutrient supplementation

Micronutrient deficiencies, often referred to as "hidden hunger," are widespread among malnourished children and must be addressed during treatment. Children with SAM are frequently deficient in vitamin A, zinc, iron, folate, and other essential nutrients. WHO guidelines recommend routine supplementation of vitamin A and folic acid during inpatient care, along with zinc supplementation for children with diarrhea to reduce the duration of diarrheal episodes. Iron supplementation is introduced only during the rehabilitation phase, once infections have been addressed, to avoid exacerbating pathogen growth [30].

In settings with high population-level deficiencies, mass supplementation strategies may be employed. These include vitamin A supplementation every six months for children under 5 years, as well as multiple micronutrient powders (MNPs) that can be added to home-cooked meals. Iron-folic acid supplementation for pregnant and lactating women is also critical to prevent intrauterine growth retardation and low birth weight, both of which increase the risk of postnatal malnutrition [39].

6.4 Preventive public health intervention strategies

Prevention of malnutrition extends beyond the health sector and requires cross-sectoral collaboration. Nutrition-specific interventions, such as therapeutic feeding, are essential but alone are insufficient to sustainably reduce malnutrition. Nutrition-sensitive interventions aim to address the underlying and basic causes of malnutrition, including poverty, food insecurity, poor sanitation, and limited maternal education, which create an enabling environment for long-term impact.

Key interventions include:

- **Nutrition education program:** This program empowers caregivers, communities, and adolescents with the knowledge needed to make informed decisions about feeding, hygiene, and health. In many low-resource settings, inadequate infant and young child feeding practices (IYCF), including early cessation of breastfeeding, delayed introduction of complementary foods, or reliance on nutrient-poor diets, are significant contributors to malnutrition [29]. Education programs should promote exclusive breastfeeding for the first 6 months, timely and appropriate complementary feeding from 6 to 23 months, and continued breastfeeding up to 2 years and beyond.

Effective approaches include community dialog, mother support groups, home visits, and mass media campaigns. Targeting both mothers and influential family members (e.g. fathers, grandmothers) enhances impact. Integrating nutrition education into antenatal care, immunization visits, and school curricula ensures broader and sustained outreach. Studies show that when mothers receive regular counseling on IYCF, rates of stunting and wasting decrease significantly.

- **Health system integration and promotion**: Integrating nutrition into primary healthcare systems is essential for early detection, referral, and preventive support [40]. Health workers at the frontline, including nurses, midwives, and community health volunteers, should be trained to provide growth monitoring and promotion (GMP), IYCF counseling, and micronutrient supplementation as part of routine child health services.

- **Growth monitoring and promotion:** GMP involves regular weight and height assessments of children under five, plotted on growth charts, and followed by counseling and action. GMP helps detect early growth faltering before it progresses to moderate or severe malnutrition. When integrated into child welfare clinics, immunization days, and community outreach, it ensures continuity of care. The integration also allows for timely identification of high-risk children, support for low-birth-weight infants, and linkage to food supplementation programs where needed [41].

- **WASH interventions:** These interventions are central to the prevention of malnutrition by breaking the infection-malnutrition cycle through the promotion of safe drinking water, hand washing, and sanitation infrastructure[42]. Poor access to safe water, open defecation, and inadequate hygiene increase the risk of diarrheal diseases and environmental enteric dysfunction (EED), a subclinical condition that impairs nutrient absorption and immune function [43]. Improving access to clean water through protected wells, piped supplies, and water purification solutions reduces waterborne disease transmission. Promoting hand washing with soap, especially before feeding and after defecation, is one of the most cost-effective interventions to reduce diarrheal episodes. In addition, improved sanitation infrastructure (e.g. latrines, community toilets) and hygiene education campaigns must be scaled up in informal settlements, refugee camps, and rural communities [44].

Programs that integrate WASH with nutrition, such as combining hygiene education with IYCF counseling or providing hygiene kits during food distributions, have shown improved child health outcomes. WHO and UNICEF emphasize WASH-Nutrition integration as essential to achieving the SDGs on health, nutrition, and water [42].

6.5 Social protection and food security

Social protection programs act as a buffer against poverty-driven malnutrition by improving household food access, caregiving capacity, and resilience. School feeding programs, implemented in over 100 countries, provide free or subsidized meals to children, improving school attendance, reducing short-term hunger, and offering a platform for micronutrient fortification[45]. In food-insecure settings, school meals can be the most consistent source of nutrition for vulnerable children [46].

Food security interventions help stabilize household access to diverse, nutritious foods. These may include food vouchers, agricultural training, seed distribution, or cash transfer programs. Linking nutrition with livelihood support helps families withstand economic shocks and reduce reliance on emergency aid [. Cash transfer programs, whether unconditional or conditional, have gained prominence as tools to reduce food insecurity and improve dietary diversity. When well-targeted, these programs empower families to buy nutritious food, reduce the need for child labor, and improve maternal mental health. Conditional transfers linked to health check-ups or school attendance promote service uptake while improving nutrition outcomes. Evidence from Latin America and SSA shows that well-designed cash transfers can reduce stunting and improve birth weights [47].

Other forms of social protection include food vouchers, public works programs, and agricultural support schemes for female-headed households. Linking these with nutrition education and health services can enhance their effectiveness and ensure long-term impact[47].

These strategies are particularly effective when implemented together, reinforcing both biological and social resilience to malnutrition.

6.6 Humanitarian coordination: Cluster approach and sphere standards

Effective nutrition interventions in emergencies require coordinated action across multiple sectors and organizations to ensure effective nutrition responses. The cluster approach, introduced by the Inter-Agency Standing Committee (IASC), designates UNICEF as the lead for the global nutrition cluster (GNC) in emergencies. The GNC ensures that humanitarian actors collaborate on needs assessments, supply chain logistics, monitoring, and technical guidance. At the country level, nutrition clusters coordinate government agencies, UN bodies, NGOs, and donors to avoid duplication, ensure equitable service delivery, and monitor performance indicators [48].

The sphere standards serve as the global benchmark for humanitarian response, outlining minimum standards for nutrition in emergencies. These include benchmarks for GAM prevalence, minimum daily energy and protein requirements, therapeutic feeding coverage, and acceptable cure and mortality rates. Adherence to sphere standards ensures accountability, quality, and effectiveness, especially in complex emergencies involving displacement, food insecurity, or disease outbreaks [43].

Together, these treatment and intervention strategies provide a comprehensive roadmap to combat childhood malnutrition. A combination of facility-based care, decentralized community programs, micronutrient support, and preventive public health strategies, anchored in coordinated humanitarian action, can significantly reduce the burden of malnutrition and improve long-term child health outcomes.

7. Monitoring, evaluation, and policy recommendations

Effective management of childhood malnutrition requires robust systems for monitoring, evaluation, and policy integration. Monitoring and evaluation (M&E)

help ensure program quality, guide decision-making, and facilitate accountability for stakeholders. Key performance indicators include recovery rates, mortality rates, defaulter rates, coverage rates, and relapse frequency. These indicators are routinely tracked in both CMAM and facility-based settings.

National and sub-national nutrition surveillance systems, such as District Health Information Software 2 (DHIS2) and rapid nutrition assessment tools (e.g. SMART surveys), enable timely data collection, trend analysis, and identification of priority areas for intervention. However, challenges remain in data quality, completeness, and real-time reporting due to infrastructure limitations, workforce shortages, and fragmented systems. In humanitarian contexts, mobile data platforms and mHealth innovations are increasingly used to support M&E efforts. Integrated dashboards that combine nutrition, WASH, and food security indicators provide a comprehensive picture of malnutrition drivers and intervention effectiveness. Regular evaluations are essential for adjusting program strategies and enhancing outcomes.

In low-resource settings and conflict-affected areas, M&E efforts face additional constraints due to insecurity, lack of infrastructure, workforce shortages, and restricted access to affected populations. Data collection may be intermittent or paper-based, with limited digital access or internet connectivity [49]. In such environments, simplified monitoring tools, such as manual tally sheets, paper-based MUAC screening logs, and sentinel site surveillance, remain essential. Community-based volunteers often serve as frontline data collectors, despite receiving minimal training. Conflict zones may also lack centralized nutrition information systems, making regional coordination and third-party monitoring crucial. Donor agencies and NGOs often support rapid assessments and real-time alerts using mobile technologies like RapidPro or KoboToolbox, which are adapted for low-bandwidth environments.

Policy implementation in these fragile settings must be flexible, allowing for emergency nutrition programming outside national systems while still aligning with core standards, such as the Sphere Minimum Standards. Governments and humanitarian actors must coordinate closely to ensure continuity of care during displacement, integrate nutrition into emergency health packages, and protect essential child health services from collapsing during crises.

On the policy side, governments should integrate nutrition into national development plans, prioritize domestic financing for nutrition programs, and strengthen multisectoral coordination among ministries of health, education, agriculture, and social welfare. Community engagement, political will, and donor support remain critical drivers of long-term impact.

8. Conclusion

Addressing childhood malnutrition requires a multidimensional and integrated strategy that encompasses clinical treatment, community-based care, preventive interventions, and coordinated emergency response. Combining facility-based protocols with community outreach and multisectoral partnerships ensures timely diagnosis, effective treatment, and long-term resilience. Prioritizing nutrition within national health policies, investing in community health systems, and aligning with global standards can significantly reduce child malnutrition and improve survival and developmental outcomes.

Conflict of interest

The authors declare no conflicts of interest.

Author details

Sumayya S. Mussa[1*] and Hadia R. Mruma[2]

1 Department of Anaesthesia and Critical Care, Ijitimai District Hospital, Ministry of Health Zanzibar, Zanzibar, Tanzania

2 Department of Anaesthesia and Critical care, St-Benedict-Ndanda Hospital, Mtwara, Tanzania

*Address all correspondence to: smussa932@gmail.com

References

[1] Govender I, Rangiah S, Kaswa R, Nzaumvila D. Malnutrition in children under the age of 5 years in a primary health care setting. The South African Family Practice. 2021;**63**(1). DOI: 10.4102/safp.v63i1.5337

[2] UNICEF, WHO, WORLD BANK. Level and trend in child malnutrition. The World Health Organization. Published online. 2023:4. Available from: https://www.who.int/publications/i/item/9789240073791

[3] Black RE, Victora CG, Walker SP, et al. Maternal and child undernutrition and overweight in low-income and middle-income countries. The Lancet. 2013;**382**(9890):427–451. DOI: 10.1016/S0140-6736(13)60937-X

[4] Muthoifin, Masithoh, Qqyi A, Nuha. *Hunger hotspots fao – wfp early warnings june to october 2024 outlook*; 2024

[5] Madewell ZJ, Keita AM, Das PMG, et al. Contribution of malnutrition to infant and child deaths in Sub-Saharan Africa and South Asia. BMJ Global Health. 2024;**9**(12). DOI: 10.1136/bmjgh-2024-017262

[6] Bhutta ZA, Das JK, Rizvi A, et al. Evidence-based interventions for improvement of maternal and child nutrition: What can be done and at what cost? The Lancet. 2013;**382**(9890): 452–477. DOI: 10.1016/S0140-6736(13)60996-4

[7] Preventing and controlling micronutrient deficiencies in populations affected by an emergency. **1**:5–6

[8] Dipasquale V, Cucinotta U, Romano C. 2020. Acute malnutrition in children: Pathophysiology, clinical effects and treatment. Nutrients. **12**(8):1–9. DOI: 10.3390/nu12082413

[9] Victora CG, Adair L, Fall C, et al. Maternal and child undernutrition: Consequences for adult health and human capital. The Lancet. 2008;**371** (9609):340–357. DOI: 10.1016/S0140-6736(07)61692-4

[10] Scaling Up Nutrition Movement. SUN 3.0: A strategy to accelerate nutrition action and systemic change, 2021–2025. Published online 2021:1–48

[11] Atukunda P, Eide WB, Kardel KR, Iversen PO, Westerberg AC. Unlocking the potential for achievement of the un sustainable development goal 2 – 'zero hunger' – In Africa: Targets, strategies, synergies and challenges. Food and Nutrition Research. 2021;**65**:1–11. DOI: 10.29219/fnr.v65.7686

[12] United Nation. *Global Nutrition Report 2021*. 2021. https://globalnutritionreport.org/documents/851/2021_Global_Nutrition_Report_aUfTRv0.pdf [Accessed: 2025-September-21]

[13] Wali N, Agho KE, Renzaho AMN. 2020. Factors associated with stunting among children under 5 years in five south asian countries (2014–2018): Analysis of demographic health surveys. Nutrients. **12**(12):1–27. DOI: 10.3390/nu12123875

[14] Net F Conflict, high prices, and below-average harvests are driving increased humanitarian needs: key messages outlook by country. 2024

[15] IPC Global Partners. Ipc Acute Food Insecurity. 2024;(September

2024):1–30. Available from: https://www.ipcinfo.org/ipcinfo-website/ipc-overview-and-classification-system/ipc-acute-food-insecurity-classification/en/

[16] Homeida A. 2023. The complexities of conflict-induced severe malnutrition in Sudan. BMJ Global Health. **8**(12):1–4. DOI: 10.1136/bmjgh-2023-014152

[17] Harghandiwal B. 2025. Impact of the humanitarian crisis in Gaza on children's health: evidence and recommendations for mitigation. Global Public Health. **20**(1):1–20. DOI: 10.1080/17441692.2025.2495326

[18] UNICEF, WHO, Bank W. UNICEF, WHO, The World BANK. Levels and Trends in Child Malnutrition, Joint Child Malnutrition Estimates 2020 Edition. 2020. Published online 2020:1–15

[19] United Nations Children's Fund Nigeria. Malnutrition rates in children under 5 years. 2015;(Mics 2011):1–9. Available from: http://www.unicef.org/nigeria/media/1646/file/%20Nigeria-equity-profile-nutrition.pdf.pdf [Accessed: 2025-September-18]

[20] Ethiopian Public Health Institute (EPHI), ICF. *Ethiopia Mini Demographic and Health Survey 2019: Final Report*. 2021. Available from: https://dhsprogram.com/pubs/pdf/FR363/FR363.pdf [Accessed: 2025-August-20]

[21] Lynch Cecelia. Humanitarian Action. In: Nord Peace Quest. Published online. 2024:165–178. DOI: 10.4324/9781003319115-11

[22] United Republic of Tanzania. United Republic of Tanzania Prime Minister's office. Published online 2021

[23] Period R, Appeal U. Humanitarian Situation UNICEF'S Response and Funding Status Situation Overview & Humanitarian Needs. 2023. Published; [Accessed: 2025-September-18]

[24] Nutrition | UNICEF Middle East and North Africa. https://www.unicef.org/mena/nutrition [Accessed: 2025-September-18]

[25] WFP. Acute malnutrition threatens half of children under five in Yemen in 2021: UN. World Food Program. Published online. 2021. Available from: https://www.wfp.org/news/acute-malnutrition-threatens-half-children-under-five-yemen-2021-un

[26] Surveillance D, Response O Whole of Syria (Wos) Monthly Situation Report. 2023; (September):2022–2023

[27] UNHCR. Using data modelling to predict displacement crises. 2023; (March). www.drc.ngo

[28] United Nations Higher Commissioner for Refugees. Global trends in forced. Published online 2024:1–48. Available from: https://www.unhcr.org/global-trends [Accessed: 2025-September-18]

[29] Matee N, Ageru TA, Mangi E, Nguyen HT, Walugembe F. Caregivers' perceptions of factors influencing undernutrition among under five in Ubungo, Dar es Salaam, Tanzania. BMC Pediatrics. 2024;**24**(1). DOI: 10.1186/s12887-024-05239-3

[30] WHO. Guidelines for the management of common childhood illnesses. *WHO Libr Cat Data World*. Published online 2013:125–143

[31] Yakubu T, Apprey C, Annan RA. Exploring current barriers and enablers of severe acute malnutrition management

among children (6–59 months): Perspectives from health professionals in northern Ghana. BMC Nutrition. 2025;**11**(1). DOI: 10.1186/s40795-025-01075-5

[32] Bliss JR, Njenga M, Stoltzfus RJ, Pelletier DL. 2016. Stigma as a barrier to treatment for child acute malnutrition in M arsabit County, Kenya. Maternal and Child Nutrition. **12**(1):125–138. DOI: 10.1111/mcn.12198

[33] Nemerimana M, Karambizi AC, Umutoniwase S, et al. Evaluation of an mHealth tool to improve nutritional assessment among infants under 6 months in paediatric development clinics in rural Rwanda: Quasi-experimental study. Maternal and Child Nutrition. 2021;**17**(4):1–12. DOI: 10.1111/mcn.13201

[34] Majiwa PR, Chopera P, Matsungo TM. Family-led mid-upper arm circumference (FL-MUAC) approach and the screening of acute malnutrition in children aged 6 to 59 months in Africa: A scoping review. Pan African Medical Journal. 2024;49. DOI: 10.11604/pamj.2024.49.38.36956

[35] Lu Z, O'Dell D, Srinivasan B, et al. Rapid diagnostic testing platform for iron and Vitamin A deficiency. the Proceedings of the National Academy of Sciences of the United States of America. 2017;**114**(51):13513–13518. DOI: 10.1073/pnas.1711464114

[36] Renzaho AMN, Dachi G, Ategbo E, Chitekwe S, Doh D. Pathways and approaches for scaling - up of community - based management of acute malnutrition programs through the lens of complex adaptive systems in South Sudan. Archives of Public Health. Published online. 2022:1–21. DOI: 10.1186/s13690-022-00934-y

[37] Chapter 8 psychosocial aspects of chapter 8 : Psychosocial aspects of.: 154–176

[38] WHO 9 april . Mental health and psychosocial well–being among children in severe food shortage situations. The International Journal of Psychology. 2006;**13**(4):333–342. Available from: http:who.int/publications/i/item/WHO-MSD-MER-06.1

[39] Rahman M, Abe SK, Rahman S, et al. Maternal anemia and risk of adverse birth and health outcomes in low- and middle-income countries : Systematic review and meta analysis. The American Journal of Clinical Nutrition. 2016;**103**:495–504. Published online. DOI: 10.3945/ajcn.115.107896

[40] Kraef C, Wood B, Philipsborn P Von, Singh S, Peterson S. & practice Primary health care and nutrition. 2020:886–893

[41] Kebede GG, Dawed YA, Seid KA. Child growth monitoring and promotion practice and associated factors among health care workers at public health facilities in south Wollo Zone, Northeast Ethiopia : A facility-based cross-sectional study. BMC Nutrition. 2022;**8**:1–13. Published online. DOI: 10.1186/s40795-022-00597-6

[42] Choi HS, Ha SY, Cha SH, Kang CG, Kim BM Design of channel type indirect blank holder for prevention of wrinkling and fracture in hot stamping process. *AIP Conf Proc*. 2011;**1383**:895–902. DOI: 10.1063/1.3623700

[43] Sphere S. *The Sphere Handbook Arabic* 2018 Fourth edition, (Geneva, Switzerland: Practical Action Publishing), 2018. DOI: 10.3362/9781908176738

[44] Global W, March P, and Note G. Nutrition-sensitive water supply, sanitation, and hygiene: Water Global Practice March 2019 guidance note. 2019. www.worldbank.org/gwsp [Accessed: 2025-September-21]

[45] Bliznashka L, Elsabbagh D, Kurdi S, Ecker O, Gelli A. 2024. School feeding for improving child nutrition in conflict-affected settings: Feasibility and cost efficiency of alternative models in Yemen. Annals of the New York Academy of Sciences. **1540**(1):251–264. DOI: 10.1111/nyas.15222

[46] Bouterakos M, Doura M, Hambayi M, and Bundy D. The importance of school feeding programmes to support the nutrition of school-age children, particularly during the COVID-19 pandemic. Field Exchange - Emergency Nutrition Network ENN. 2021;**66**:12–14. Available from: https://www.ennonline.net/sites/default/files/FEX-66-Final-(2)_12-14.pdf

[47] Tiwari S, Daidone S, Ruvalcaba MA, et al. Impact of cash transfer programs on food security and nutrition in Sub-Saharan Africa: A cross-country analysis. Glob Food Sec. 2016;**11** (10):72–83. DOI: 10.1016/j.gfs.2016.07.009

[48] IASC. Guidance; Cluster Coordination at country level- IASC Sub-Working Group on the Cluster Approach and the Global Cluster Coordinators' Group. 2018(July). Available from: https://interagencystandingcommittee.org/iasc-transformative-agenda/iasc-reference-module-cluster-coordination-country-level-revised-july-2015

[49] Challenges of doing M&E in FCV settings _ Better Evaluation

Section 2

Neonatal Sepsis and Survival

Chapter 2

Global Trends in Neonatal Sepsis: A Scopus Bibliometric Analysis of Publications from 2015 to 2025

Festus Mulakoli

Abstract

Neonatal sepsis remains a significant global health challenge, contributing to substantial morbidity and mortality, particularly in low- and middle-income countries (LMICs). This bibliometric study aimed to analyze research trends, key contributors, emerging themes, and collaborative networks in the neonatal sepsis literature from 2015 to mid-2025. The Scopus database was searched using relevant keywords. After applying the inclusion and exclusion criteria, the final dataset was analyzed using bibliometric methods. The annual publication trend showed a steady growth from 2015 to 2020. The United States, China, and India were the top contributors, while the University of Toronto, St. George's University of London, and Inserm are leading institutions. Keyword co-occurrence analysis revealed clusters around biomarkers, maternal health, and antimicrobial resistance. Collaboration networks highlighted strong partnerships among high-income countries but limited integration with high-burden regions. Key research gaps include the need for context-specific diagnostic tools, capacity building in LMICs, and understanding the long-term outcomes of neonatal sepsis survivors. This study emphasizes the urgent need for equitable research investments, strengthened global partnerships, and targeted interventions to reduce the burden of neonatal sepsis, particularly in regions with the highest disease burden.

Keywords: neonatal sepsis, early-onset sepsis (EOS), late-onset sepsis (LOS), septicemia, neonatal mortality

1. Introduction

Neonatal sepsis is a systemic infection that occurs in newborns within the first 28 days of life and is characterized by the presence of bacteria, viruses, or fungi in the bloodstream, leading to systemic inflammatory response syndrome (SIRS) [1]. It is classified as early-onset sepsis (EOS), occurring within 72 hours of birth, or late-onset sepsis (LOS), developing after 72 hours, with EOS typically acquired vertically from the mother and LOS often associated with hospital-acquired infections [2]. Its clinical presentation is often nonspecific and may include temperature instability, respiratory distress (e.g., grunting and apnea), feeding intolerance, lethargy, irritability, hypotension, and signs of poor perfusion [2]. Severe cases can progress to septic shock, disseminated intravascular coagulation (DIC), and multi-organ failure, necessitating prompt diagnosis and treatment to reduce mortality and long-term complications [3].

Neonatal sepsis remains a significant global health challenge, contributing to neonatal morbidity and mortality, particularly in low- and middle-income countries (LMICs). It is a life-threatening condition caused by systemic infections in newborns and typically occurs within the first 28 days of life. Despite advances in neonatal care, the burden of neonatal sepsis persists due to factors such as antimicrobial resistance (AMR), limited access to quality healthcare, and inadequate infection prevention practices [4].

Neonatal sepsis remains a leading cause of morbidity and mortality worldwide, particularly in LMICs where healthcare resources are limited. Globally, an estimated three million cases of neonatal sepsis occur annually, accounting for 11% of all neonatal deaths and approximately 500,000 fatalities each year [4]. The burden is disproportionately high in sub-Saharan Africa and South Asia, where access to healthcare, hygiene, and maternal health services is often inadequate [5–7].

EOS accounts for a considerable proportion of LMIC cases due to intrapartum infections, whereas LOS is more common in neonatal intensive care units (NICUs), particularly among preterm and exceptionally low-birth-weight infants [8]. Survivors of neonatal sepsis experience long-term complications, including neurodevelopmental impairment, growth retardation, and increased susceptibility to recurrent infections, further straining the healthcare system [5]. Addressing neonatal sepsis requires improved maternal healthcare, infection prevention strategies, and timely antibiotic administration to reduce its global burden.

According to the World Health Organization (WHO), sepsis is responsible for approximately 15% of all neonatal deaths globally, with an estimated three million cases of neonatal sepsis occurring annually. The burden is disproportionately higher in sub-Saharan Africa and South Asia, where healthcare systems often struggle with resource constraints and delayed diagnosis. WHO's global report on the epidemiology and burden of sepsis emphasizes the urgent need for improved surveillance, prevention strategies, and research to address this critical health issue [6].

Neonatal sepsis exhibits significant regional disparities, with the highest incidence and mortality rates observed in LMICs, owing to limited healthcare access, poor sanitation, and inadequate maternal and neonatal care. Globally, the incidence of neonatal sepsis is estimated at 2,200 cases per 100,000 live births; however, in sub-Saharan Africa and South Asia, the rate is 5,000–7,500 per 100,000 live births, which is three to five times higher than that in high-income countries (HICs) [4]. In South Asia, countries such as India, Pakistan, and Bangladesh report sepsis in 15%–20% of hospitalized neonates, with case fatality rates exceeding 25% in rural settings [7]. Similarly, in sub-Saharan Africa, neonatal sepsis accounts for 30%–50% of neonatal deaths, with incidence rates peaking in regions with high rates of premature birth, unhygienic deliveries, and maternal infections [9]. In contrast, HICs, such as those in the United States and Western Europe, report much lower rates (500–1,000 per 100,000 live births), which is attributed to sterile delivery practices, widespread antenatal care, and advanced neonatal intensive care [1]. These stark disparities highlight the urgent need for targeted interventions in LMICs, including maternal immunization, clean birth practices, and improved antibiotic stewardship to reduce preventable neonatal deaths.

Neonatal sepsis remains a significant cause of morbidity and mortality worldwide, and multiple interrelated factors influence its development. Maternal conditions play a crucial role, as prolonged membrane rupture (> 18 hours) significantly increases the risk of ascending infections [10]. Maternal infections, including chorioamnionitis, urinary tract infections, and Group B Streptococcus (GBS) colonization, are strongly associated with early-onset neonatal sepsis [11, 12]. This risk is particularly elevated in preterm infants, whose immature immune systems and underdeveloped physiological barriers make them exceptionally vulnerable to systemic infections [13].

The circumstances surrounding delivery constitute another category of critical risk factor. Unsterile delivery practices, common in resource-limited settings, dramatically increase exposure to potential pathogens [14]. Complications such as meconium-stained amniotic fluid and prolonged labor have been independently associated with higher rates of neonatal sepsis [10]. Invasive procedures, including instrumental deliveries and frequent vaginal examinations, further compound this risk by introducing additional opportunities for bacterial contamination [1]. These findings underscore the importance of skilled birth attendance and appropriate infection-control measures during delivery.

Neonatal characteristics significantly influence susceptibility to sepsis. Low birth weight (< 2,500 g) and prematurity are among the strongest predictors, with the risk being inversely proportional to gestational age and birth weight [15]. Hospitalized neonates face additional hazards, such as prolonged NICU stays, invasive devices, and mechanical ventilation, which increase their exposure to nosocomial pathogens [16, 17]. The protective effect of breastfeeding has been well-documented, with formula-fed infants demonstrating higher rates of infection owing to the absence of maternal immunoglobulins and other protective factors in breast milk [1, 18]. These risk factors highlight the need for targeted preventive strategies to reduce the global burden of neonatal sepsis among high-risk populations.

Accurate epidemiological data collection for neonatal sepsis faces numerous challenges, particularly in low-resource settings where the burden is the highest. Diagnostic limitations represent a major barrier, as the clinical signs of sepsis are nonspecific and overlap with those of other neonatal conditions [19]. Blood culture, the gold standard for diagnosis, has low sensitivity (30%–50%) in neonates because of the small blood volumes obtained and frequent antibiotic pretreatment [7]. In low-income countries, limited laboratory infrastructure and inflated costs prevent routine culture testing, leading to reliance on clinical diagnosis alone, which lacks specificity [9].

Inconsistent case definitions across studies and surveillance systems further complicate the comparability of data. While some programs use WHO clinical criteria, others incorporate laboratory markers or treatment responses, creating heterogeneity in the reported incidence rates [4]. Underreporting is widespread, especially in community settings, where many sepsis-related deaths occur without medical attention. Hospital-based surveillance misses these cases, whereas verbal autopsies, used as substitutes, have questionable accuracy [20].

Health system challenges, including fragmented record-keeping, paper-based systems, and incomplete mortality registries, have led to data gaps [21]. Security issues and geographical barriers prevent the enumeration of cases in conflict and remote areas [22]. Even in high-income settings, variations in sepsis coding (ICD-10 [International Classification of Diseases, tenth revision] versus clinical criteria) affect surveillance accuracy [23–25].

Addressing these challenges requires standardized definitions, improved diagnostics, and investment in health information systems. Novel approaches, such as machine learning algorithms for risk prediction and biomarker panels, may enhance future surveillance [26]. Until then, global sepsis estimates represent a significant underestimation of the true burden.

Despite the high burden and clinical significance of neonatal sepsis, research is fragmented and unevenly distributed across regions and disciplines. Neonatal sepsis remains one of the leading causes of neonatal mortality, accounting for approximately 203,000 deaths annually and affecting an estimated 1.3 million neonates globally each year [27]. The burden is disproportionately higher in LMICs, particularly in sub-Saharan Africa and South Asia [28].

A systematic review and meta-analysis found that data on neonatal sepsis incidence and mortality are limited and highly variable, especially in resource-limited settings, complicating global comparisons and policy planning [29]. According to the Global Burden of Disease Study 2019, the global incidence of neonatal sepsis increased by 12.79% from 1990 to 2019, while mortality decreased by 12.93%, indicating some progress but also highlighting persistent challenges [30].

There is a lack of comprehensive understanding of how the scientific community has addressed neonatal sepsis over the past decade, which topics have been prioritized, which countries and institutions have led the research, and how collaborative networks have evolved. This gap hinders the ability of policymakers, clinicians, and researchers to identify knowledge deficits, effectively allocate resources, and foster global cooperation. The WHO and other global health bodies have emphasized the urgent need for coordinated research efforts and investment in neonatal infection surveillance and prevention strategies.

Bibliometric analysis is a powerful tool for systematically mapping the landscape of scientific literature and uncovering trends, influential publications, key contributors, and emerging research themes [31]. By analyzing publications from 2015 to 2025, this study aimed to provide a decade-long overview of neonatal sepsis research. This analysis is crucial for identifying research hotspots and gaps to guide future investigations, highlighting global and regional contributions to fostering equitable research development, understanding collaboration patterns to strengthen international partnerships, and informing funding agencies and policymakers regarding strategic investment areas. This bibliometric study will serve as a foundational resource for stakeholders to enhance their global response to neonatal sepsis through evidence-based strategies and coordinated research.

Neonatal sepsis is a critical public health concern owing to its high mortality rate, long-term complications, and substantial economic burden on healthcare systems, particularly in low-resource settings. As a leading cause of neonatal death, it contributes significantly to global under-five mortality, hindering progress toward the United Nations Sustainable Development Goal (SDG) 3.2, which aims to reduce preventable newborn deaths. Survivors often face neurodevelopmental delays, growth impairments, and increased susceptibility to infections, leading to lifelong disabilities that strain families and healthcare infrastructure [4]. Its economic impact is profound, with prolonged hospitalization, intensive care needs, and escalating antibiotic resistance treatment costs [32]. Addressing neonatal sepsis requires strengthening maternal and neonatal healthcare systems, promoting infection prevention measures, ensuring timely antibiotic access, and enhancing global surveillance. Public health interventions, such as maternal immunization, clean birthing practices, and neonatal sepsis management protocols, can significantly reduce the burden, particularly in high-risk regions. Prioritizing neonatal sepsis is essential not only for improving survival rates but also for ensuring healthier future generations and sustainable healthcare systems [33–36].

Despite advances in neonatal care, significant gaps in knowledge and practice persist regarding the prevention, diagnosis, and management of neonatal sepsis. Diagnostic uncertainty remains a critical challenge because current biomarkers, such as C-reactive protein (CRP) and procalcitonin (PCT), lack sufficient sensitivity and specificity in the early stages of infection [37]. The field urgently needs validated biomarker panels that can distinguish true sepsis from non-infectious inflammatory conditions while providing rapid, point-of-care results [38]. Additionally, the optimal duration of antibiotic therapy remains controversial, particularly in culture-negative cases, as it contributes to antimicrobial overuse and resistance [39].

A major research gap exists in population-specific sepsis definitions, as the current criteria, derived from high-income settings, may not apply to low-birthweight neonates or to resource-limited areas. The pathogenesis of sepsis in preterm infants, particularly how immature immune responses interact with specific pathogens, is poorly understood [40]. Furthermore, while maternal immunization shows promise in preventing EOS (e.g., GBS vaccines), implementation barriers in LMICs remain unaddressed [41].

Clinical practice gaps include inconsistent adoption of sepsis bundles across facilities, especially in LMICs, where staffing and resource constraints limit protocol adherence [42]. There is also inadequate evidence to guide post-sepsis neurodevelopmental follow-up, despite the known risk of long-term impairment [43]. Most critically, the intersection of sepsis and AMR in neonatal units requires innovative stewardship approaches tailored to vulnerable populations [32].

Closing these gaps demands harmonized research priorities that address both biological mechanisms and implementation science. Future research should focus on precision diagnostics, targeted immunotherapies, and context-specific prevention strategies that account for the global health disparities in neonatal care.

This study has the potential to significantly transform neonatal sepsis management by addressing critical gaps in diagnosis, treatment, and prevention. By validating novel biomarker panels for early and accurate sepsis detection, this study could reduce diagnostic delays and unnecessary antibiotic use, particularly in resource-limited settings where laboratory infrastructure is scarce [38]. The development of context-specific clinical algorithms tailored to different healthcare environments (e.g., NICUs vs. community clinics) may standardize care and improve outcomes in diverse populations [44, 45].

Investigations into optimized antibiotic regimens could lead to evidence-based guidelines on the duration and selection of antimicrobials, helping to combat rising resistance rates while maintaining treatment efficacy [39]. Furthermore, by elucidating immune–pathogen interactions in preterm infants, these findings may pave the way for targeted immunotherapies or adjuvant treatments to modulate dysregulated host responses [46].

At the public health level, research could strengthen preventive strategies such as maternal vaccination protocols or improved infection control bundles, potentially reducing the incidence of sepsis in high-risk settings [41, 47, 48]. By integrating machine learning tools for risk prediction, this study may also enable initiative-taking interventions in vulnerable neonates [49, 50].

This work could inform global guidelines, shape health policies, and reduce the burden of neonatal sepsis, particularly in LMICs, where the mortality toll is the highest. The translational impact spans from bench to bedside, offering scalable solutions to save lives and improve long-term outcomes for survivors.

2. Primary objectives

To analyze global research trends, key contributors, emerging themes, and collaborative networks in neonatal sepsis literature over the past decade (2015–2025) using bibliometric methods, providing insights into the evolution of knowledge, gaps, and future research directions.

3. Methods

3.1 Study design

This study employed a retrospective bibliometric design to analyze global research output on neonatal sepsis published between 2015 and 2025. Bibliometric techniques were used to quantitatively and qualitatively assess publication trends, authorship patterns, institutional productivity, international collaboration, and thematic evolution in the field.

3.2 Data source and search strategy

3.2.1 Database selection

Bibliometric data were extracted from Scopus, a comprehensive and widely recognized database for scholarly literature. Scopus was selected for its extensive coverage of peer-reviewed journals, robust citation tracking, and compatibility with bibliometric software.

3.2.2 Search query

A structured search strategy was developed using relevant keywords and Boolean operators to capture literature on neonatal sepsis. The final query included ("neonatal sepsis" OR "newborn sepsis" OR "infant sepsis" OR "neonatal infection") AND (diagnosis OR treatment OR management OR outcomes). This query was applied to titles, abstracts, and keywords to ensure comprehensive retrieval of relevant publications.

3.2.3 Inclusion and exclusion criteria

3.2.3.1 Inclusion criteria

To ensure the relevance and quality of the bibliometric analysis, the study included peer-reviewed publications such as original research articles, review articles, meta-analyses, and clinical guidelines that directly contribute to neonatal sepsis research. Publications such as conference abstracts, editorials, letters, case reports, and non-English articles (unless deemed critical) were excluded to maintain methodological rigor. An initial search in Scopus yielded 6,088 records, which were imported into EndNote X20 for deduplication using automated and manual methods. Titles and abstracts were screened for relevance, and full-text reviews were conducted for borderline cases.

3.2.3.2 Exclusion criteria

Specific exclusion criteria were applied during the screening process to ensure the relevance and quality of the dataset. Publications such as conference abstracts, editorials, letters to the editor, and case reports were excluded because of their limited methodological rigor and lack of comprehensive data. Additionally, non-English language articles were excluded unless they were deemed critical to the field, particularly if they addressed unique regional challenges or contributed significantly to the discourse on neonatal sepsis.

3.2.4 Bibliometric analysis

3.2.4.1 Quantitative metrics

To assess the evolution of neonatal sepsis research over the past decade, annual publication trends were analyzed to identify patterns of growth and fluctuations in scholarly output. Citation metrics, including total citations, average citations per year, and author h-index, were evaluated to determine the impact and influence of individual researchers, journals, and articles within the field.

3.2.4.2 Network analysis

To explore patterns of scholarly collaboration and intellectual influence in neonatal sepsis research, country and institutional partnerships were visualized using VOSviewer (v.1.6.20). These collaboration networks highlight the key global research hubs and cross-national linkages. Additionally, author co-citation analysis was conducted to identify influential researchers and thematic clusters, revealing the intellectual structure and leading contributors shaping the field over the past decade.

3.2.4.3 Keyword and thematic analysis

To identify the dominant research themes in the neonatal sepsis literature, a keyword co-occurrence analysis was conducted. Keywords were extracted from the dataset and clustered using bibliometric tools, revealing major thematic areas such as AMR, biomarker-based diagnostics, and maternal-neonatal health. These clusters reflect the evolving research priorities and highlight the interdisciplinary nature of neonatal sepsis research.

3.2.4.4 Statistical and visualization tools

Descriptive statistics, primarily counts and percentages, were used to summarize the publication and citation data. Analytical outputs and visualizations were generated using VOSviewer for network mapping and Microsoft Excel for tabular and graphical representations, ensuring the clarity and accessibility of the bibliometric findings.

4. Ethical considerations

This study relied exclusively on publicly available metadata and did not involve human participants, identifiable personal data, or interventions. Therefore, ethical approval was not required for this study.

5. Results

Based on an initial Scopus search, 6,088 records were retrieved and screened. After applying the inclusion and exclusion criteria, a final dataset of 6,088 articles was retained for bibliometric analysis.

5.1 Annual publication trend

Figure 1 shows that between 2014 and mid-2025, the volume of publications on neonatal sepsis exhibited a dynamic trajectory, reflecting evolving research priorities and global health concerns. The number of studies increased steadily from 359 in 2015 to 781 in 2020. However, the subsequent years showed fluctuations, and by 2024, the number of publications had dropped significantly to approximately 368.

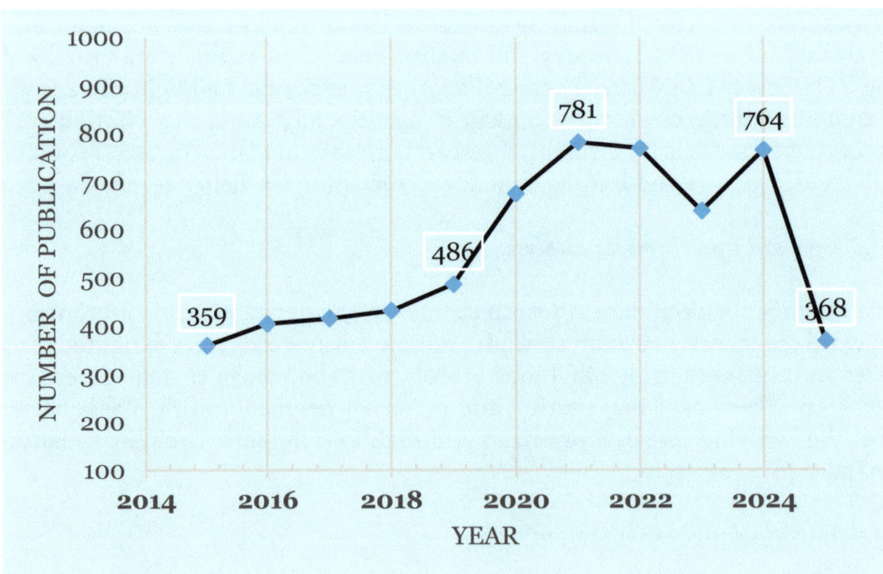

Figure 1.
Trends in neonatal sepsis research publications (2015–2025): a decade of research output.

5.2 Country/Institution

Bibliometric analysis revealed that the United States leads neonatal sepsis research output, contributing 1,290 publications, followed by China (n = 625) and India (n = 598). These three countries collectively account for a significant portion of global research in this domain. Other notable contributors include the United Kingdom (n = 502), Italy (n = 288), and Australia (n = 269), as shown in **Table 1**.

At the institutional level (see **Table 2**), the University of Toronto ranks highest, with 83 publications, closely followed by St. George's, University of London (n = 77), and the Institut National de la Santé et de la Recherche Médicale (Inserm; n = 75). Prestigious institutions, such as Harvard Medical School (n = 71), The Children's Hospital of Philadelphia (n = 74), and the University of Oxford (n = 64), also feature prominently. European institutions include Université Paris Cité (n = 65), Erasmus MC (n = 67), and AP–HP Assistance Publique-Hôpitaux de Paris (n = 67).

Country	Publications
United States	1,290
China	625
India	598
United Kingdom	502
Italy	288
Australia	269
Canada	261
Turkey	216
The Netherlands	214
France	200

Table 1.
Countries with the highest number of publications in neonatal sepsis in last ten years (2015–2025).

Institutions	Publications
University of Toronto	83
St George's, University of London	77
Inserm	75
The Children's Hospital of Philadelphia	74
Harvard Medical School	71
London School of Hygiene & Tropical Medicine	69
AP–HP Assistance Publique – Hôpitaux de Paris	67
Erasmus MC	67
Université Paris Cité	65
University of Oxford	64

Table 2.
Top 10 institutions contributing to neonatal sepsis research output in last ten years (2015–2025).

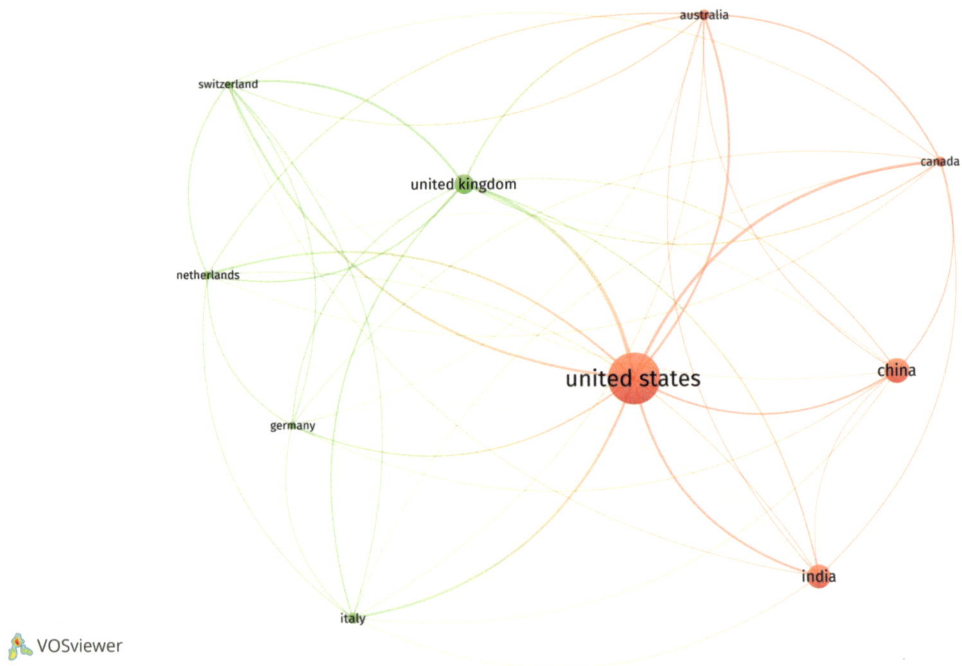

Figure 2.
Global collaboration network in neonatal sepsis research (2015–2025): Top 10 country-level co-authorship trends. The size of the node represents the number of publications that the countries have collaborated to author.

5.3 Collaboration between countries

Figure 2 illustrates the collaborative network of international partnerships in neonatal sepsis research. Two main clusters were identified in the VOSviewer analysis (green and red). The United States stands out as a central hub, forming strong collaborative ties with countries such as India, Canada, and Australia, as represented by the green cluster. By contrast, the United Kingdom has a collaborative network with Germany, Italy, Switzerland, the Netherlands, and Sweden, as represented by the red cluster. Other collaboration networks are observed between the United States and the United Kingdom, the United States and Switzerland, and the United States and the Netherlands. In addition, there is collaboration between the United Kingdom, Australia, and Canada.

5.4 Author co-citation and co-authorship network analysis

As shown in **Figure 3**, the authors' co-citation network revealed key influencers and thematic clusters in neonatal sepsis research. Two clusters were identified (red and green), with prominent researchers such as Wyse, Stoll, Puopolo, and Romero, who had a high frequency of co-citations.

Co-authorship network analysis (see **Figure 4**) revealed two prominent clusters of researchers actively collaborating in the field of neonatal sepsis. The red cluster, which includes authors such as Hansen M., Stoll J., Wynn J.L., Puopolo K.M., and Polin R.A., and, on the other side, the green cluster, features authors like Romero R. and Yoon B.H.

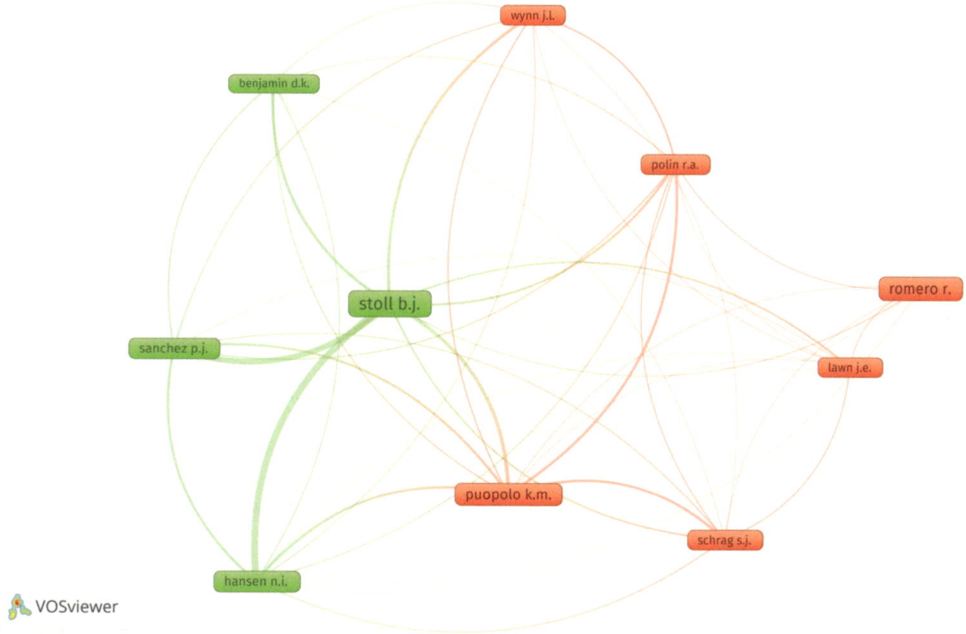

Figure 3.
Global Co-citation network among authors conducting studies on neonatal sepsis research between 2015 and 2025. Each node represents an author, and two authors are considered to have co-citation if their papers are frequently cited together.

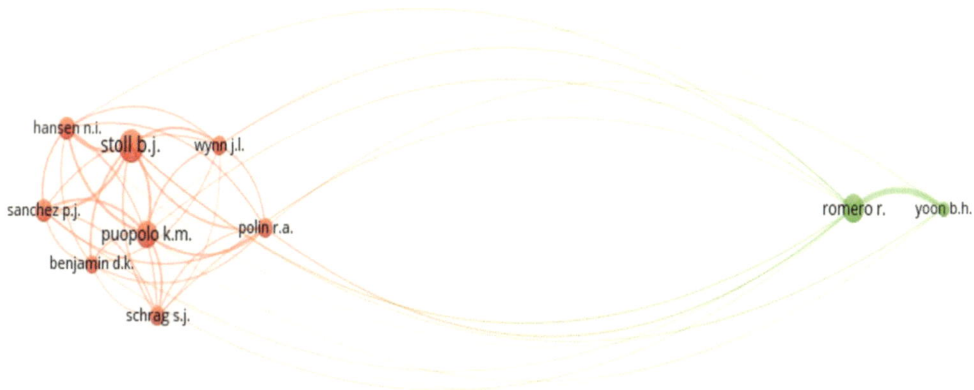

Figure 4.
Global Co-authorship network among top10authors in neonatal sepsis research (2015–2025). Each node represents an author, and a link between two nodes indicates that the authors have co-authored publications together

5.5 Co-occurrence analysis

The co-occurrence analysis of keywords, as shown in **Figure 5**, revealed three major thematic clusters (green, red, and blue) in neonatal sepsis research. The green cluster includes terms such as "sepsis," "neonate," and "infection," representing foundational concepts and general clinical focus areas in neonatal sepsis; the red cluster contains keywords like "neonatal sepsis," "pregnancy," and "antibiotics"; and the blue cluster features keywords such as "procalcitonin" and "C-reactive protein."

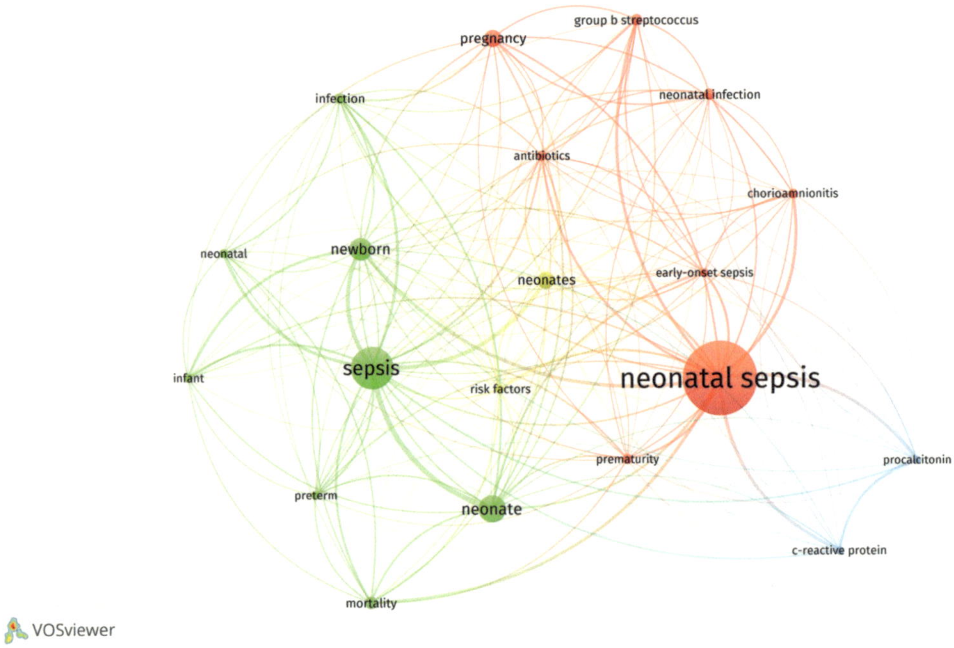

Figure 5.
Top 20 keyword co-occurrence network analysis as used by authors in neonatal sepsis research (2015–2025). The thickness of the connecting lines reflects the strength of association betweeb keywords, while the size and color intensity of the circles indicates the frequency of keywords occurence in publications

6. Discussion

This bibliometric study presents a comprehensive overview of neonatal sepsis research over the past decade, revealing key patterns in publication output, international collaboration, thematic evolution, and scholarly influence. The findings yield several important insights with significant implications for global health policy and the prioritization of research [51].

The steady increase in annual publications from 2015 to 2020, culminating in a peak in 2020, reflects the growing global recognition of neonatal sepsis as a significant public health concern. The pronounced spike in 2020 was correlated with the COVID-19 pandemic, which intensified the focus on infectious disease pathogenesis, immune responses, and neonatal vulnerabilities. The subsequent decline by 2024 may indicate a post-pandemic reallocation of research priorities or temporary saturation in certain thematic areas, underscoring the need for a renewed focus on persistent and emerging challenges, particularly AMR and rapid diagnostic innovation [52, 53].

A central finding is the stark disparity between research output and the disease burden. The dominance of HICs, particularly the United States, the United Kingdom, and China, in publication volume and institutional productivity underscores the profound imbalance in global research capacity. This is a well-documented phenomenon in global health literature, often referred to as the "10/90 gap," where only a fraction of research resources address the health problems of the majority of the world's population [54]. Consequently, regions with the highest burden of neonatal sepsis, namely sub-Saharan Africa and South Asia, remain critically underrepresented in scholarly literature. This misalignment emphasizes the urgent ethical and practical imperative for equitable investment in research infrastructure, sustainable funding, and local capacity building in LMICs [55].

Despite having the highest burden of neonatal sepsis and mortality globally, African institutions have contributed minimally to publication volume. This aligns with epidemiological data confirming that sub-Saharan Africa has the highest neonatal mortality rate due to sepsis, which is often exacerbated by limited access to diagnostics and antibiotics [56]. The Global Burden of Disease study further affirms that Africa has the highest disability-adjusted life years (DALYs) related to neonatal sepsis; however, its bibliometric visibility remains disproportionately low [57]. This gap underscores the pressing need for targeted regional investment and ethically informed North–South and South–South collaborations [58].

India and China have emerged as major contributors, with a combined output of over 1,200 publications. This is consistent with the data showing that South Asia has the highest absolute number of neonatal sepsis cases. The thematic focus from India, as identified in our keyword analysis, heavily emphasizes AMR and empirical antibiotic use, reflecting local challenges with multidrug-resistant pathogens. However, the literature consistently highlights systemic barriers, such as antibiotic overuse and a lack of standardized, cost-effective diagnostic protocols [59].

In Europe and North America, the United States, United Kingdom, and European nations such as Italy and France reflect their established research infrastructure and funding. Institutions such as Harvard University and the University of Oxford are frequently cited for their leadership in developing consensus definitions, advancing biomarker validation, and conducting large-scale clinical trials [60, 61]. The strong intra-regional collaboration networks observed mirror EU-funded initiatives, such as the NeoVanc and PERFORM consortia, which focus on optimizing treatment and diagnostics. The low neonatal sepsis mortality rates in these regions are attributed to advanced neonatal intensive care and robust surveillance systems [62, 63].

The Eastern Mediterranean and Latin America, which have seen rising sepsis burdens, have demonstrated a modest but growing research output. Studies from countries such as Iran, Egypt, and Brazil have often focused on maternal risk factors, environmental exposure, and health system resilience [64–66]. Our keyword analysis identified clusters around "pregnancy" and "infection," aligning with the regional focus on perinatal care and EOS [67]. However, limited data harmonization and international collaboration continue to hinder comprehensive regional assessments.

Co-citation analysis confirms the foundational influence of a core group of researchers (e.g., Stoll B.J., Puopolo K.M., and Romero R.), whose work on diagnostics, risk stratification, and maternal–fetal immunology has established current clinical standards. The clustering of authors suggests distinct yet interconnected intellectual communities driving subfields such as immunology, microbiology, and clinical epidemiology.

One of the most striking novel findings of this analysis is the emergence of a dense, highly focused research cluster around biomarkers, particularly PCT and CRP, which were not as prominent in earlier decades [68, 69]. This signifies a paradigm shift toward precision diagnostics, aiming to move beyond subjective clinical signs to enable earlier, more accurate detection [70]. The implications for LMICs are significant. If validated as a cost-effective point-of-care tool in these settings, such biomarkers could drastically reduce antibiotic overuse and improve survival rates [71].

Furthermore, the network analyses clearly identified robust collaboration within HICs but limited the integration of high-burden regions. This presents a clear strategic opportunity: fostering targeted, equitable partnerships between high-output and high-burden regions could accelerate the development and implementation of context-specific solutions, from novel diagnostics to simplified treatment algorithms. These findings underscore that transforming neonatal outcomes globally requires a triad of targeted investments in diagnostic innovation, inclusive collaborative networks, and regional research capacity-building.

Neonatal sepsis remains a significant health challenge across sub-Saharan Africa and contributes to neonatal mortality in this region. Neonatal infections, including sepsis, account for approximately 26% of neonatal deaths annually, with sub-Saharan Africa having one of the highest mortality rates globally [28]. Despite the global decline in neonatal mortality rates, sepsis continues to be a major impediment, particularly in this region [72].

Several risk factors have been identified in sub-Saharan Africa that exacerbate the burden of neonatal sepsis. These include low birth weight, prematurity, low Apgar scores, male sex, prolonged rupture of membranes, and intrapartum fever [56]. Socioeconomic factors, such as low socioeconomic status and rural residence, also contribute to an increased risk of neonatal sepsis [73]. The economic burden is substantial, with estimates suggesting a loss of 5.29 to 8.73 million DALYs annually due to neonatal sepsis in the region, translating to an economic burden of $10 billion to $469 billion [28].

Efforts to mitigate this burden include improving antenatal care utilization to identify and manage risk factors effectively and implementing WHO-recommended interventions, which have the potential to significantly reduce neonatal mortality from sepsis and other related conditions [72, 74]. An enhanced focus on recognizing and managing pre-existing conditions that increase neonatal vulnerability, such as acute kidney injury, hypothermia, and asphyxia, may also help reduce the incidence and severity of neonatal sepsis [75]. Despite these efforts, there is a critical need for increased investment in high-quality research and healthcare strategies specifically tailored to the sub-Saharan context to improve outcomes and address the substantial burden of neonatal sepsis across the region [73].

Neonatal sepsis poses a significant global health challenge, with substantial implications for both morbidity and mortality in newborns. Globally, an estimated 6.31 million incident cases of neonatal sepsis occur annually, with approximately 0.23 million deaths attributed to this condition [76]. This burden is most pronounced in LMICs, where sepsis accounts for a substantial proportion of neonatal deaths [23]. A key factor exacerbating the burden of neonatal sepsis is the emergence of multidrug-resistant pathogens, particularly in regions with limited health care resources. For instance, *Acinetobacter* spp., a common pathogen in neonatal sepsis, is often resistant to first-line treatments recommended by the WHO, complicating treatment efforts [77]. Similarly, *Klebsiella pneumoniae*, another leading pathogen, shows increasing resistance to multiple antibiotics, including meropenem, posing a significant threat as AMR continues to increase [78].

Efforts to mitigate this burden include preventive strategies such as maternal vaccination against pathogens like *Klebsiella pneumoniae*, which models suggest could significantly reduce the incidence of neonatal sepsis and associated mortality. Such vaccinations could potentially avert over 80,000 neonatal deaths and 400,000 sepsis cases annually worldwide, particularly in Africa and Southeast Asia [78].

Despite advances in medical research, challenges persist in accurately diagnosing and managing neonatal sepsis, contributing to variations in global estimates of the sepsis burden [79]. Innovations in diagnostic biomarkers, such as heparin-binding protein (HBP), may offer promise in the early detection and management of the disease, potentially improving in-hospital outcomes [80]. The global incidence of neonatal sepsis has been increasing; however, mortality rates have shown a declining trend owing to improved healthcare interventions [76]. Continuous efforts to enhance healthcare delivery, increase awareness, and implement targeted interventions remain crucial for addressing the global burden of neonatal sepsis. Although we could not generate a full essay, the information provided offers a comprehensive overview of the global burden of neonatal sepsis based on the available literature.

6.1 Strengths and limitations

A key strength of this bibliometric analysis lies in its comprehensive scope, covering a full decade (2015–2025) of neonatal sepsis research across multiple dimensions, including publication trends, author influence, institutional productivity, international collaboration, and thematic focus. The integration of co-authorship, co-citation, and keyword co-occurrence analyses provides a multi-layered understanding of the field's intellectual structure and evolution. Additionally, the study's alignment with global regions allows for a contextual interpretation of research output relative to disease burden, offering valuable insights for policy and funding decisions.

However, this study has some limitations. First, it relies on citation-based metrics, which may not fully capture the clinical impact or real-world relevance of research, especially in low-resource settings where publication rates are lower. Second, the analysis may be affected by database coverage bias, as some regional and non-English publications are underrepresented on major indexing platforms. Third, the sharp decline in publications by 2024 may reflect a data lag rather than an actual drop in research activity. Finally, while collaboration networks were mapped, the study did not assess the quality or outcomes of these partnerships, which is crucial for translating research into practice.

6.2 Clinical and public health implications

The findings of this bibliometric analysis have significant implications for both clinical practice and public health policy. The increasing focus on biomarkers, such as PCT and CRP, suggests a shift toward early and more precise diagnosis of neonatal sepsis, which could reduce reliance on empirical antibiotic therapy and help curb AMR, a major global health threat. The identification of regional disparities in research output, particularly the underrepresentation of high-burden regions such as sub-Saharan Africa and South Asia, highlights the need for equitable resource allocation and capacity building in neonatal care. Strengthening surveillance systems, improving access to diagnostics, and fostering international collaboration are essential steps toward reducing neonatal mortality. Moreover, the clustering of research on maternal health and infection control underscores the importance of integrated perinatal care strategies that address both maternal and neonatal risk factors. These insights can inform targeted interventions, guideline development, and funding priorities to globally improve outcomes in neonates.

The findings of this bibliometric study have important implications for shaping public health policies and designing targeted interventions to combat neonatal sepsis. The clear disparity between regions with a high disease burden and low research output, particularly in sub-Saharan Africa and parts of South Asia, highlights the urgent need for policy-driven investments in research infrastructure, surveillance systems, and clinical training in these areas. Governments and global health organizations should prioritize funding for context-specific diagnostic tools, such as biomarker-based assays, which have shown promise in the recent literature and are prominent in this study's thematic clusters. Furthermore, the strong collaboration networks observed among HICs suggest that international partnerships can be leveraged to support capacity-building and knowledge transfer in underrepresented regions.

Public health policies should also incorporate findings from influential research clusters, such as those focused on antimicrobial stewardship and maternal–neonatal health, to develop integrated care models that address both prevention and early treatment. Aligning research priorities with public health needs can lead to more equitable and effective strategies to reduce neonatal sepsis-related mortality worldwide.

7. Conclusion

This bibliometric analysis of neonatal sepsis research from 2015 to 2025 reveals a decade of dynamic scholarly activity, marked by increasing publication trends, evolving thematic priorities, and expanding global collaboration. The findings underscore the central role of HICs in driving research output and shaping intellectual discourse, while also highlighting the underrepresentation of regions with the highest disease burden, such as sub-Saharan Africa and South Asia. The emergence of biomarker-focused studies and maternal–neonatal health themes reflects a shift toward precision diagnostics and integrated care approaches. Strong co-authorship and co-citation networks indicate influential researchers and institutions that have guided the development of the field. However, disparities in research capacity and collaboration underscore the need for inclusive, equitable global partnerships. This study provides a valuable roadmap for future research, policy formulation, and clinical innovation aimed at reducing the global impact of neonatal sepsis.

8. Future directions

The results of this bibliometric analysis indicated several promising avenues for future research on neonatal sepsis. First, the growing emphasis on biomarker-based diagnostics, such as PCT and CRP, calls for multicenter validation studies, especially in low-resource settings where early diagnosis could significantly reduce mortality. Second, the observed regional disparities in research output highlight the need for studies that explore context-specific risk factors, care practices, and microbial profiles in underrepresented regions such as sub-Saharan Africa and Southeast Asia. Third, the limited integration between high-output and high-burden regions suggests a need for research on models of equitable collaboration, including capacity-building frameworks and knowledge-sharing platforms. Additionally, future studies should investigate the long-term neurodevelopmental outcomes of neonatal sepsis survivors, an area that remains underexplored despite its importance to public health. Finally, the emergence of machine learning and predictive analytics in neonatal care presents an opportunity to develop and evaluate AI-driven decision-support tools for early sepsis detection and management. These directions can help bridge the existing gaps and enhance the global response to neonatal sepsis.

Author details

Festus Mulakoli
School of Nursing and Midwifery, Aga Khan University, Nairobi, Kenya

*Address all correspondence to: mulakolifesto@gmail.com

References

[1] Shane AL, Sánchez PJ, Stoll BJ. Neonatal sepsis. The Lancet. 2017;**390** (10104):1770–1780

[2] Zeigler AC, Ainsworth JE, Fairchild KD, Wynn JL, Sullivan BA. Sepsis and mortality prediction in very low birth weight infants: Analysis of HeRO and nSOFA. American Journal of Perinatology. 2023;**40**(4):407–414.

[3] Sturrock S, Ali S, Gale C, Battersby C, Le Doare K. Neonatal outcomes and indirect consequences following maternal SARS-CoV-2 infection in pregnancy: A systematic review. BMJ Open. 2023;**13**(3):e063052

[4] Fleischmann-Struzek C, Goldfarb DM, Schlattmann P, Schlapbach LJ, Reinhart K, Kissoon N. The global burden of paediatric and neonatal sepsis: A systematic review. The Lancet Respiratory Medicine. 2018;**6**(3):223–230

[5] Wynn JL, Polin RA. A neonatal sequential organ failure assessment score predicts mortality to late-onset sepsis in preterm very low birth weight infants. Pediatric Research. 2020;**88** (1):85–90

[6] Wen SCH, Ezure Y, Rolley L, Spurling G, Lau CL, Riaz S, Paterson DL, Irwin AD. Gram-negative neonatal sepsis in low- and lower-middle-income countries and WHO empirical antibiotic recommendations: A systematic review and meta-analysis. PLOS Medicine. 2021;**18**(9):e1003787

[7] Sankar MJ, Natarajan CK, Das RR, Agarwal R, Chandrasekaran A, Paul VK. When do newborns die? A systematic review of timing of overall and cause-specific neonatal deaths in developing countries. Journal of Perinatology. 2016;**36**(Suppl 1):S1–s11

[8] Zozaya C, García González I, Avila-Alvarez A, Oikonomopoulou N, Sánchez Tamayo T, Salguero E, de Pipaón M S, García-Muñoz Rodrigo F, Couce ML. Incidence, Treatment, and Outcome Trends of Necrotizing Enterocolitis in Preterm Infants: A Multicenter Cohort Study. Frontiers in Pediatrics. 2020;**8**:188

[9] Seale AC, Obiero CW, Berkley JA. Rational development of guidelines for management of neonatal sepsis in developing countries. Current Opinion in Infectious Diseases. 2015;**28**(3): 225–230. https://www.ncbi.nlm.nih.gov/pubmed/25887615

[10] Pergialiotis V, Bellos I, Antsaklis A, Papapanagiotou A, Loutradis D, Daskalakis G. Maternal and neonatal outcomes following a prolonged second stage of labor: A meta-analysis of observational studies. European Journal of Obstetrics & Gynecology and Reproductive Biology. 2020;**252**:62–69

[11] Zou H, Jia X, He X, Su Y, Zhou L, Shen Y, Sheng C, Liao A, Li C, Li Q. Emerging threat of multidrug resistant pathogens from neonatal sepsis. Frontiers in Cellular and Infection Microbiology. 2021;**11**:694093

[12] Yahya FB, Hathcock MA. A retrospective review of neonatal sepsis among GBS-Colonized women undergoing planned cesarean section after labor onset or rupture of membranes. Infectious Diseases in

Obstetrics and Gynecology. 2020;**2020**:4365259

[13] Fanaroff AA, Fanaroff JM. Advances in Neonatal Infections. American Journal of Perinatology. 2020;**37**(S 02):S5–s9

[14] Yohannes D, Manilal A, Woldemariam M, Aklilu A, Zakir A, Batire S, Negede B, Alodaini HA, Idhayadhulla A. Bacterial profile, antibiotic susceptibility patterns and associated factors among neonates suspected of omphalitis in Arba Minch, Southern Ethiopia. Scientific Reports. 2025;**15**(1):14404

[15] Zeng S, Liu Y, Chen M, Ruan T, Lu W, Liu X. Timing of intravenous prophylactic antibiotic agents for cesarean delivery: A systematic review and meta-analysis of randomized controlled trials. Surgical Infections. 2023;**24**(4):303–310

[16] Su Z, Gao M, Weng L, Xu T. Esculin targets TLR4 to protect against LPS-induced septic cardiomyopathy. International Immunopharmacology. 2024;**131**:111897

[17] Bonger ZT, Mamo BT, Birra SB, Yalew AW. Predictors of length of hospital stay for preterm infants in Ethiopia: A competing risk analysis. Frontiers in Pediatrics. 2023;**11**:1268087

[18] Carbone F, Montecucco F, Sahebkar A. Current and emerging treatments for neonatal sepsis. Expert Opinion on Pharmacotherapy. 2020;**21**(5):549–556

[19] Wynn JL. Defining neonatal sepsis. Current Opinion in Pediatrics. 2016;**28**(2):135–140

[20] Lona-Reyes JC, Miramontes-Buiza L, Frías-Flores LF, Regla-Nava JA, González-Carmona J, Gallegos-Marín JA, Chávez-Rodríguez M. Risk factors associated with neonatal sepsis due to Serratia marcescens in a public hospital in Mexico: A case-control study. 2025. DOI: 10.1016/j.ram.2025.04.006

[21] Dietz BW, Jones TK, Small DS, Gaieski DF, Mikkelsen ME. The relationship between index hospitalizations, sepsis, and death or transition to hospice care during 30-day hospital readmissions. Medical Care. 2017;**55**(4):362–370

[22] Gupta V, Pandita A, Panghal A, Pillai A. Leucocyte adhesion defect presenting as fulminant sepsis in a new born. BMJ Case Reports. 2019;**12**(8):e227065

[23] Zaka N, Alexander EC, Manikam L, Norman ICF, Akhbari M, Moxon S, Ram PK, Murphy G, English M, Niermeyer S, Pearson L. Quality improvement initiatives for hospitalised small and sick newborns in low- and middle-income countries: A systematic review. Implementation Science. 2018;**13**(1):20

[24] Sands K, Spiller OB, Thomson K, Portal EAR, Iregbu KC, Walsh TR. Early-onset neonatal sepsis in low- and middle-income countries: Current challenges and future opportunities. Infection and Drug Resistance. 2022;**15**:933–946

[25] Rhee C, Dantes R, Epstein L, Murphy DJ, Seymour CW, Iwashyna TJ, Kadri SS, Angus DC, Danner RL, Fiore AE, Jernigan JA, Martin GS, Septimus E, Warren DK, Karcz A, Chan C, Menchaca JT, Wang R, Gruber S, Klompas M. Incidence and

trends of sepsis in US hospitals using clinical vs claims data, 2009-2014. Jama. 2017;**318**(13):1241–1249

[26] Zhang J, Xu X, Wang M. Clinical significance of serum miR-101-3p expression in patients with neonatal sepsis. Personalized Medicine. 2021;**18**(6):541–550

[27] Li J, Xiang L, Chen X, Li S, Sun Q, Cheng X, Hua Z. Global, regional, and national burden of neonatal sepsis and other neonatal infections, 1990-2019: Findings from the global burden of disease study 2019. European Journal of Pediatrics. 2023;**182**(5):2335–2343

[28] Ranjeva SL, Warf BC, Schiff SJ. Economic burden of neonatal sepsis in sub-Saharan Africa. BMJ Global Health. 2018;**3**(1):e000347

[29] Zelellw DA, Dessie G, Worku Mengesha E, Balew Shiferaw M, Mela MM, Emishaw S. A systemic review and meta-analysis of the leading pathogens causing neonatal sepsis in developing countries. BioMed Research International. 2021;**2021**:6626983

[30] Zhang Y, Li S, Li Y, Zheng J, Dong Y. Analysis and risk factors of deep vein catheterization-related bloodstream infections in neonates. Medicine (Baltimore). 2024;**103**(12): e37184

[31] Kumar R. Bibliometric analysis: Comprehensive insights into tools, techniques, applications, and solutions for research excellence. Spectrum of Engineering and Management Sciences. 2025;**3**(1):45–62

[32] Laxminarayan R, Matsoso P, Pant S, Brower C, Røttingen JA, Klugman K, Davies S. Access to effective antimicrobials: A worldwide challenge. The Lancet. 2016;**387**(10014):168–175

[33] Lassi ZS, Fisher Z, Andraweera P, Cummins A, Roberts CT. Effectiveness of birthing kits for clean childbirth: A systematic review. International Health. 2020;**12**(1):3–10

[34] Gon G, Ali SM, Towriss C, Kahabuka C, Ali AO, Cavill S, Dahoma M, Faulkner S, Haji HS, Kabole I, Morrison E, Said RM, Tajo A, Velleman Y, Woodd SL, Graham AWJ. Unpacking the enabling factors for hand, cord and birth-surface hygiene in Zanzibar maternity units. Health Policy and Planning. 2017;**32**(8):1220–1228

[35] Vekemans J, Crofts J, Baker CJ, Goldblatt D, Heath PT, Madhi SA, Le Doare K, Andrews N, Pollard AJ, Saha SK, Schrag SJ, Smith PG, Kaslow DC. The role of immune correlates of protection on the pathway to licensure, policy decision and use of group B Streptococcus vaccines for maternal immunization: Considerations from World Health Organization consultations. Vaccine. 2019;**37**(24):3190–3198

[36] Zea-Vera A, Ochoa TJ. Challenges in the diagnosis and management of neonatal sepsis. Journal of Tropical Pediatrics. 2015;**61**(1):1–13. https://www.ncbi.nlm.nih.gov/pubmed/25604489

[37] Pontrelli G, De Crescenzo F, Buzzetti R, Jenkner A, Balduzzi S, Calò Carducci F, Amodio D, De Luca M, Chiurchiù S, Davies EH, Copponi G, Simonetti A, Ferretti E, Di Franco V, Rasi V, Della Corte M, Gramatica L, Ciabattini M, Livadiotti S, Rossi P. Accuracy of serum procalcitonin for the diagnosis of sepsis in neonates and children with systemic inflammatory

syndrome: A meta-analysis. BMC Infectious Diseases. 2017;**17**(1):302

[38] Wynn JL, Polin RA. Progress in the management of neonatal sepsis: The importance of a consensus definition. Pediatric Research. 2018;**83**(1):13–15

[39] Cantey JB, Anderson KR, Kalagiri RR, Mallett LH. Morbidity and mortality of coagulase-negative staphylococcal sepsis in very-low-birth-weight infants. World Journal of Pediatrics. 2018;**14**(3):269–273

[40] Raturi A, Chandran S. Neonatal sepsis: Aetiology, pathophysiology, diagnostic advances and management strategies. Clinical Medicine Insights: Pediatrics. 2024;**18**:11795565241281337

[41] Sorano S, Procter SR, Seale AC. Cost-effectiveness analysis of maternal vaccination against Group B streptococcus in Japan. Vaccine: X. 2023;**14**:100332

[42] Sands K, Carvalho MJ, Spiller OB, Portal EAR, Thomson K, Watkins WJ, Mathias J, Dyer C, Akpulu C, Andrews R, Ferreira A, Hender T, Milton R, Nieto M, Zahra R, Shirazi H, Muhammad A, Akif S, Jan MH, Iregbu K, Modibbo F, Uwaezuoke S, Chan GJ, Bekele D, Solomon S, Basu S, Nandy RK, Naha S, Mazarati JB, Rucogoza A, Gaju L, Mehtar S, Bulabula ANH, Whitelaw A, Walsh TR. Characterisation of staphylococci species from neonatal blood cultures in low- and middle-income countries. BMC Infectious Diseases. 2022;**22**(1):593

[43] Stoll BJ, Puopolo KM, Hansen NI, Sánchez PJ, Bell EF, Carlo WA, Cotten CM, D'Angio CT, Kazzi SNJ, Poindexter BB, Van Meurs KP, Hale EC, Collins MV, Das A, Baker CJ, Wyckoff MH, Yoder BA, Watterberg KL, Walsh MC, Devaskar U, Laptook AR, Sokol GM, Schrag SJ, Higgins RD. Early-onset neonatal sepsis 2015 to 2017, the rise of escherichia coli, and the need for novel prevention strategies. JAMA Pediatrics. 2020;**174**(7):e200593

[44] Ackermann K, Baker J, Festa M, McMullan B, Westbrook J, Li L. Computerized clinical decision support systems for the early detection of sepsis among pediatric, neonatal, and maternal inpatients: Scoping review. JMIR Medical Informatics. 2022;**10**(5):e35061

[45] Eisenberg M, Madden K, Christianson JR, Melendez E, Harper MB. Performance of an automated screening algorithm for early detection of pediatric severe sepsis. Pediatric Critical Care Medicine. 2019;**20**(12):e516–e23

[46] Polcz VE, Rincon JC, Hawkins RB, Barrios EL, Efron PA, Moldawer LL, Larson SD. Trained Immunity: A potential approach for improving host immunity in neonatal sepsis. Shock. 2023;**59**(2):125–134

[47] Russell LB, Kim SY, Cosgriff B, Pentakota SR, Schrag SJ, Sobanjo-Ter Meulen A, Verani JR, Sinha A. Cost-effectiveness of maternal GBS immunization in low-income sub-Saharan Africa. Vaccine. 2017;**35**(49):6905–6914

[48] Prasad PA, Shea ER, Shiboski S, Sullivan MC, Gonzales R, Shimabukuro D. Relationship between a sepsis intervention bundle and in-hospital mortality among hospitalized patients: A retrospective analysis of real-world data. Anesthesia & Analgesia. 2017;**125**(2):507–513

[49] van den Berg Mam, Medina O, Loohuis IIP, van der Flier Mm, Dudink JJ, Benders M, Bartels RRT, Vijlbrief DDC, van den Berg MAM, van der Flier MM. Development and clinical impact assessment of a machine-learning model for early prediction of late-onset sepsis. Computers in Biology and Medicine. 2023;**163**:107156

[50] Meyer MP, Alexander T. Reduction in necrotizing enterocolitis and improved outcomes in preterm infants following routine supplementation with Lactobacillus GG in combination with bovine lactoferrin. Journal of Neonatal-Perinatal Medicine. 2017;**10**(3):249–255

[51] Gańczak M, Miazgowski T, Kożybska M, Kotwas A, Korzeń M, Rudnicki B, Nogal T, Andrei CL, Ausloos M, Banach M, Brazinova A, Constantin MM, Dubljanin E, Herteliu C, Hostiuc M, Hostiuc S, Jakovljevic M, Jozwiak JJ, Kissimova-Skarbek K, Król ZJ, Mestrovic T, Miazgowski B, Milevska Kostova N, Naghavi M, Negoi I, Negoi RI, Pana A, Rubino S, Sekerija M, Sierpinski R, Szponar L, Topor-Madry R, Vujcic IS, Widecka J, Widecka K, Wojtyniak B, Zadnik V, Kopec JA. Changes in disease burden in Poland between 1990-2017 in comparison with other Central European countries: A systematic analysis for the Global Burden of Disease Study 2017. PLoS One. 2020;**15** (3):e0226766

[52] Sharma M, Jain M, Veeraraghavan B, Rodrigues C, Bansal N, Nambi PS, Nangia S, Singhal T, Walia K. Target product profiles for diagnosis of sepsis: Proposing a new approach for diagnostic innovation. Indian Journal of Medical Research. 2023;**157**(5):395–402

[53] Curtin SC, Tejada-Vera B, Bastian BA. Deaths: Leading causes for 2020. National Vital Statistics Reports: From the Centers for Disease Control and Prevention, National Center for Health Statistics, National Vital Statistics System. 2023;**72**(13):1–115

[54] Kilama WL. The 10/90 gap in sub-Saharan Africa: Resolving inequities in health research. Acta Tropica. 2009 ; **112**:S8–S15. https://www.sciencedirect.com/science/article/pii/S0001706X09002447

[55] Woods WA, Watson M, Ranaweera S, Tajuria G, Sumathipala A. Under-representation of low and middle income countries (LMIC) in the research literature: Ethical issues arising from a survey of five leading medical journals: Have the trends changed? Global Public Health. 2023;**18** (1):2229890

[56] Bech CM, Stensgaard CN, Lund S, Holm-Hansen C, Brok JS, Nygaard U, Poulsen A. Risk factors for neonatal sepsis in Sub-Saharan Africa: A systematic review with meta-analysis. BMJ Open. 2022;**12**(9):e054491

[57] Ni M, Zhou J, Hu M, Zhou W, Yuan T. Global, regional, and national burden of neonatal infectious diseases from 1990 to 2021. Translational Pediatrics. 2025;**14**(7):1498–1510

[58] Molloy EJ, Wynn JL, Bliss J, Koenig JM, Keij FM, McGovern M, Kuester H, Turner MA, Giannoni E, Mazela J, Degtyareva M, Strunk T, Simons SHP, Janota J, Plotz FB, van den Hoogen A, de Boode W, Schlapbach LJ, Reiss IKM. on behalf of the Infection II, Immunisation section of the E. Neonatal sepsis: Need for consensus definition, collaboration and core outcomes. Pediatric Research. 2020;**88**(1):2–4.

https://www.ncbi.nlm.nih.gov/pubmed/32193517

[59] Agarwal S, Patodia J, Mittal J, Singh Y, Agnihotri V, Sharma V. Antibiotic stewardship in a tertiary care NICU of northern India: A quality improvement initiative. BMJ Open Quality. 2021;**10**(Suppl 1):e001470

[60] Singer JR, Blosser EG, Zindl CL, Silberger DJ, Conlan S, Laufer VA, DiToro D, Deming C, Kumar R, Morrow CD, Segre JA, Gray MJ, Randolph DA, Weaver CT. Preventing dysbiosis of the neonatal mouse intestinal microbiome protects against late-onset sepsis. Nature Medicine. 2019;**25**(11):1772–1782

[61] Zhu H, Yin L, Sun Y, Xu Y, Ma J, Qiao L. Identification and validation of signature genes and their correlations with infiltrated immune cells in neonatal sepsis. Alternative Therapies in Health and Medicine. 2023;**29**(7): 272–277

[62] Hill LF, Clements MN, Turner MA, Donà D, Lutsar I, Jacqz-Aigrain E, Heath PT, Roilides E, Rawcliffe L, Alonso-Diaz C, Baraldi E, Dotta A, Ilmoja ML, Mahaveer A, Metsvaht T, Mitsiakos G, Papaevangelou V, Sarafidis K, Walker AS, Sharland M. Optimised versus standard dosing of vancomycin in infants with gram-positive sepsis (NeoVanc): A multicentre, randomised, open-label, phase 2b, non-inferiority trial. The Lancet Child & Adolescent Health. 2022;**6**(1):49–59

[63] Ericson JE, Burgoine K, Kumbakumba E, Ochora M, Hehnly C, Bajunirwe F, Bazira J, Fronterre C, Hagmann C, Kulkarni AV, Kumar MS, Magombe J, Mbabazi-Kabachelor E, Morton SU, Movassagh M, Mugamba J, Mulondo R, Natukwatsa D, Kaaya BN, Olupot-Olupot P, Onen J, Sheldon K, Smith J, Ssentongo P, Ssenyonga P, Warf B, Wegoye E, Zhang L, Kiwanuka J, Paulson JN, Broach JR, Schiff SJ. Neonatal paenibacilliosis: Paenibacillus infection as a novel cause of sepsis in term neonates with high risk of sequelae in uganda. Clinical Infectious Diseases. 2023;**77**(5):768–775

[64] Akbarian-Rad Z, Riahi SM, Abdollahi A, Sabbagh P, Ebrahimpour S, Javanian M, Vasigala V, Rostami A. Neonatal sepsis in Iran: A systematic review and meta-analysis on national prevalence and causative pathogens. PLoS One. 2020;**15**(1):e0227570

[65] Okumura MC, Aragon DC, Carvalheiro CG, Quintana SM, Mussi-Pinhata MM. High incidence rates of early-onset bacterial sepsis in infants born in two brazilian maternities: A 15-year retrospective analysis. Pediatric Infectious Disease Journal. 2024;**43**(3):271–277

[66] Seliem WA, Sultan AM. Etiology of early onset neonatal sepsis in neonatal intensive care unit - Mansoura, Egypt. Journal of Neonatal-Perinatal Medicine. 2018;**11**(3):323–330

[67] Zhou P, Zhou Y, Liu B, Jin Z, Zhuang X, Dai W, Yang Z, Feng X, Zhou Q, Liu Y, Xu X, Zhang L. Perinatal antibiotic exposure affects the transmission between maternal and neonatal microbiota and is associated with early-onset sepsis. mSphere. 2020;**5**(1):e00984-19

[68] Armstrong SJ, Brady JJ, Drew RJ, Foran A. Point-of-care procalcitonin trends in suspected neonatal late-onset infection: A prospective observational study. Pediatric Research. 2025;**97**(6):1958–1965

[69] Aggarwal S, Sangle AL, Siddiqui MS, Haseeb M, Engade MB. An observational study on C-reactive protein to platelet ratio in neonatal sepsis. Cureus. 2024;**16**(6):e62230

[70] Hofer N, Jank K, Strenger V, Pansy J, Resch B. Inflammatory indices in meconium aspiration syndrome. Pediatric Pulmonology. 2016;**51**(6): 601–606

[71] Adhisivam B. Point of care diagnostic markers for neonatal sepsis. Indian Journal of Pediatrics. 2024;**91** (6):537–538

[72] Adatara P, Afaya A, Salia SM, Afaya RA, Konlan KD, Agyabeng-Fandoh E, Agbinku E, Ayandayo EA, Boahene IG. Risk factors associated with neonatal sepsis: A case study at a specialist hospital in Ghana. The Scientific World Journal. 2019;**2019**:9369051

[73] Traoré FB, Sidibé CS, Diallo EHM, Camara BS, Sidibé S, Diallo A, Diarra NH, Ly BA, Ag Ahmed MA, Kayentao K, Touré A, Camara A, Delamou A, Sangho H, Terera I. Prevalence and factors associated with maternal and neonatal sepsis in sub-Saharan Africa: A systematic review and meta-analysis. Frontiers in Public Health. 2024;**12**:1272193

[74] Griffin JB, Jobe AH, Rouse D, McClure EM, Goldenberg RL, Kamath-Rayne BD. Evaluating WHO-Recommended interventions for preterm birth: A mathematical model of the potential reduction of preterm mortality in Sub-Saharan Africa. Global Health: Science and Practice. 2019;**7** (2):215–227

[75] Dessalegn N, Alene T, Terefe TF, Kassaw A, Genie YD, Workye H, Bimerew M. Acute kidney injury magnitude, mortality, and associated factors among neonates in sub-Saharan Africa: A systematic review and meta-analysis. Pediatric Nephrology. 2025;**40**(10):3067–3076

[76] Li J, Shen L, Qian K. Global, regional, and national incidence and mortality of neonatal sepsis and other neonatal infections, 1990-2019. Frontiers in Public Health. 2023;**11**:1139832

[77] Pillay K, Ray-Chaudhuri A, O'Brien S, Heath P, Sharland M. Acinetobacter spp. in neonatal sepsis: An urgent global threat. Frontiers in Antibiotics. 2024;**3**:1448071

[78] Kumar CK, Sands K, Walsh TR, O'Brien S, Sharland M, Lewnard JA, Hu H, Srikantiah P, Laxminarayan R. Global, regional, and national estimates of the impact of a maternal Klebsiella pneumoniae vaccine: A Bayesian modeling analysis. PLOS Medicine. 2023;**20**(5):e1004239

[79] Popescu CR, Cavanagh MMM, Tembo B, Chiume M, Lufesi N, Goldfarb DM, Kissoon N, Lavoie PM. Neonatal sepsis in low-income countries: Epidemiology, diagnosis and prevention. Expert Review of Anti-infective Therapy. 2020;**18**(5):443–452

[80] Beyzarov E, Chen Y, Caubel P. A retrospective case series analysis of pregnancy and COVID-19 based on a global postmarketing COVID-19 surveillance program. Clinical Therapeutics. 2024;**46**(7):529–537

Chapter 3

Neonatal Survival Against LMIC Odds – Case Notes of 10 Near-Death Neonates Rescued by a New Initiative

Ebenovbe Idemudia, Ann Brai and Hippolite O. Amadi

Abstract

Respiratory distress is a leading cause of neonatal mortality in low- and middle-income countries (LMICs), where access to mechanical ventilation and conventional CPAP devices remains limited, including at tertiary care levels in special care baby units (SCBUs). In response to this gap, the respiratory support substation (RespSS) initiative, a semi-detached section of the SCBU having independent assemblies of locally innovated respiratory devices, such as low-cost bubble CPAP machines, was adopted as a vital tool in the management of neonatal respiratory conditions at the University of Benin Teaching Hospital (UBTH), Nigeria. This chapter presents 10 compelling case stories of neonates managed with the RespSS during the first 12 months of use, highlighting its effectiveness in extremely low birth weight preterm neonates, infants with congenital anomalies, perinatal birth asphyxia, and severe respiratory distress syndromes. These stories not only demonstrate the technical success of the RespSS but also reflect powerful human narratives – parents overcoming infertility, survival against well-known clinical odds at UBTH, and the use of the RespSS where all other options had failed. The chapter discusses a selection of criteria, therapeutic protocols, and outcomes while exploring key themes such as innovation in low-resource settings, caregiver resilience, and the transformative role of locally adapted technologies in neonatal care. The findings underscore the urgent need to scale up RespSS-type interventions across similar healthcare systems to reduce preventable neonatal deaths and improve long-term outcomes.

Keywords: neonatal survival, LMIC, critical care outcomes, near-miss neonates, case series

1. Introduction

Neonatal mortality remains a critical public health challenge in Nigeria, with respiratory distress among the top three leading causes. The World Health Organization (WHO) reports that over one million newborns die annually from complications related to preterm birth, low birth weight, and perinatal asphyxia – many of which are preventable with timely respiratory support (WHO) [1]. In high-income countries, conventional CPAP and mechanical ventilators are standard components of neonatal intensive care. However, in many Nigerian tertiary hospitals, these technologies are often unavailable, unaffordable, or unsustainable due to erratic power supply, inadequate maintenance, and limited technical expertise. Therefore, patients are poorly managed, leading to the persistently well-known high neonatal mortality rate in Nigeria. In a recent successful collaborative effort to support measures for the improvement of neonatal care in Nigeria, an initiative was developed whereby a specially designed substation with unique respiratory support devices was introduced within an existing special care baby unit (SCBU). The respiratory support substation (RespSS) is semi-independent of the wider SCBU activities, as it is tasked with sub-admitting patients with respiratory failures and sub-discharging them back to the wider SCBU when the neonate is guided into stable, independent respiratory ability [2].

1.1 RespSS at UBTH

The SCBU of the University of Benin Teaching Hospital (UBTH), desirous of bridging this failure gap, welcomed the installation of the RespSS and the use of its locally manufactured, cost-effective continuous positive airway pressure (CPAP) system known as the PoliteHeartCPAP machine, among other locally sourced innovative systems that power the RespSS. The RespSS devices are carefully crafted to be low-cost, power-efficient, and feasible for use even in peripheral settings. Since its introduction in the neonatology unit of UBTH, the RespSS has significantly altered the course of care for critically ill neonates, especially those previously considered unsalvageable due to the lack of efficient ventilatory support.

1.2 Definition of the RespSS scope of duty

The roles of this SCBU subsection are clearly defined and exclusively designed to operate solely for these purposes, including: (i) rescuing the respiratory deterioration of the infant by completely taking over the work of effective breathing for the neonate, (2) functioning as a tool to enhance the algorithmic withdrawal of oxygen dependency for the maintenance of the neonate's physiological oxygen saturation, and (3) functioning as a tool to smoothly train the infant to achieve sustained unassisted breathing without positive end-expiratory pressure (PEEP). Neonates are referred and sub-admitted to the RespSS from the regular hall of the SCBU for this special task. Upon achieving sustained and stable independent breathing, the neonate's RespSS case is closed, and the infant is sub-discharged back into the regular SCBU hall for the continuation of treatment for other non-respiratory issues before their final discharge from the SCBU. The infant's status at the point of this sub-discharge marks the RespSS outcome for documentation. The scope of the RespSS intervention is limited to the point of sub-discharge, irrespective of the final outcome with other issues in the wider SCBU, provided the patient was sub-discharged alive and the later cause of death is not traced back to the treatment received at the RespSS. Hence, RespSS failure is established only if the neonate is confirmed to have died of respiratory failure while being treated in the RespSS. When a neonate is kept alive at the RespSS but is unable to complete the treatment course and hence gets prematurely discharged alive owing to family decisions, other compelling referral issues to other facilities, or cases of discharge-against-medical-advice (DAMA), then such a RespSS case is counted as a success at the point of discharge. RespSS outcome is not recorded as a failure when a neonate on the treatment course is confirmed to have died from another overlapping treatment, such as minor surgical procedures (e.g., line-setting) while on the PoliteHeart CPAP support.

In the 12 months of its operation since the installation and commissioning of the RespSS at UBTH, a total of 34 dire cases have been referred to the substation for support. Thirty-two of the 34 cases were successfully sub-discharged. Two died from bleeding diathesis outside the scope of the RespSS duties, and two of the infants, after discharge, passed away in the regular SCBU hall owing to other clinical reasons.

This chapter presents 10 compelling RespSS case stories among the 34 dire neonates who presented and were successfully sub-discharged in the SCBU of UBTH. These real-life narratives offer a window into the resilience of neonates and their families, the challenges of neonatal care in a resource-limited environment such as ours, and the life-saving potential of local innovations such as the RespSS. Each story goes beyond the clinical presentation to reflect the emotional and societal significance of every survival.

2. Methodology/Case selection criteria

2.1 Case selection process

The 10 cases presented in this chapter were retrospectively selected from records of 34 neonates managed in the RespSS at UBTH between September 2024 and August 2025. The inclusion criteria were based on the following:

- Clear documentation of sub-admission in the RespSS, initiation of the intervention devices, and full tracking of the algorithmized process duration.
- Presence of compelling clinical features or social abjection (e.g., extreme prematurity, survival despite severe birth asphyxia, RespSS use after other CPAP brand failures, or extraordinary family and caregiver circumstances).
- Availability of outcome data up to sub-discharge into the wider SCBU or follow-up.

2.2 Ethical considerations

Patient identities were anonymized using initials or coded identifiers. All data were de-identified to ensure confidentiality. This report does not include any personally identifiable information or photographic material. Ethical clearance was not required for this descriptive case series, which is part of internal program evaluation and knowledge sharing.

2.3 The RespSS use at UBTH

The RespSS devices (featuring: the PoliteHeart CPAP machine [3], the Politeoxygen splitter system (PSS) [4], the polite-light-bank [5], the oxygen concentrator, and the solar subpower unit and the 'rat-monitor' that secures the subpower station) were routinely used throughout the first year (September 2024 to date) of the RespSS at UBTH-SCBU (see **Figure 1** and **Figure 2**). The substation is situated in an exclusive corner of the SCBU for neonates presenting with:

- Respiratory distress syndrome (RDS);
- Recurrent apnoea of prematurity;
- Severe birth asphyxia;
- As an alternative, after other CPAP failures.

The PoliteHeart CPAP device is equipped with the capability for immediate direct pulmonary warming via patient-specific, appropriate settings of inspiratory gas temperature that achieve the physiological thermoneutral range for adequate pulmonary performance. This gives the PoliteHeart CPAP the advantage of providing immediate help to preserve the birth-transitory organic pulmonary surfactant and subsequently keeping the lungs at appropriate physiological temperatures for optimal lung performance. An earlier study showed that all neonates who maintained lower-than-physiological temperature ranges during CPAP intervention died [6]. Therefore, the treatment protocols in the RespSS typically involve early initiation of the PoliteHeart CPAP (within the first hours of life), continuous monitoring of oxygen saturation and respiratory rate, adjunctive therapies like caffeine citrate, and algorithmized gradual weaning as the clinical condition improves. Pharmaceutical surfactants were rarely administered and only

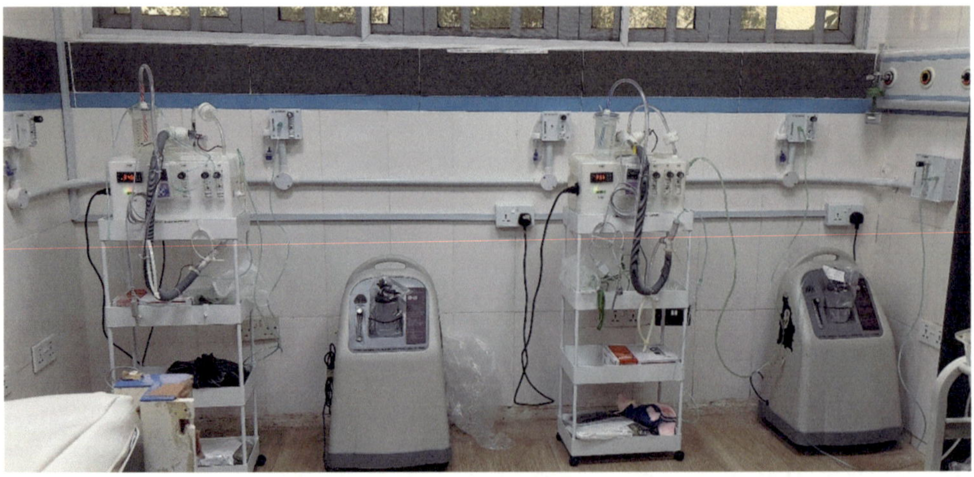

Figure 1.
The RespSS corner at the SCBU of the University of Benin Teaching Hospital (UBTH), Nigeria.

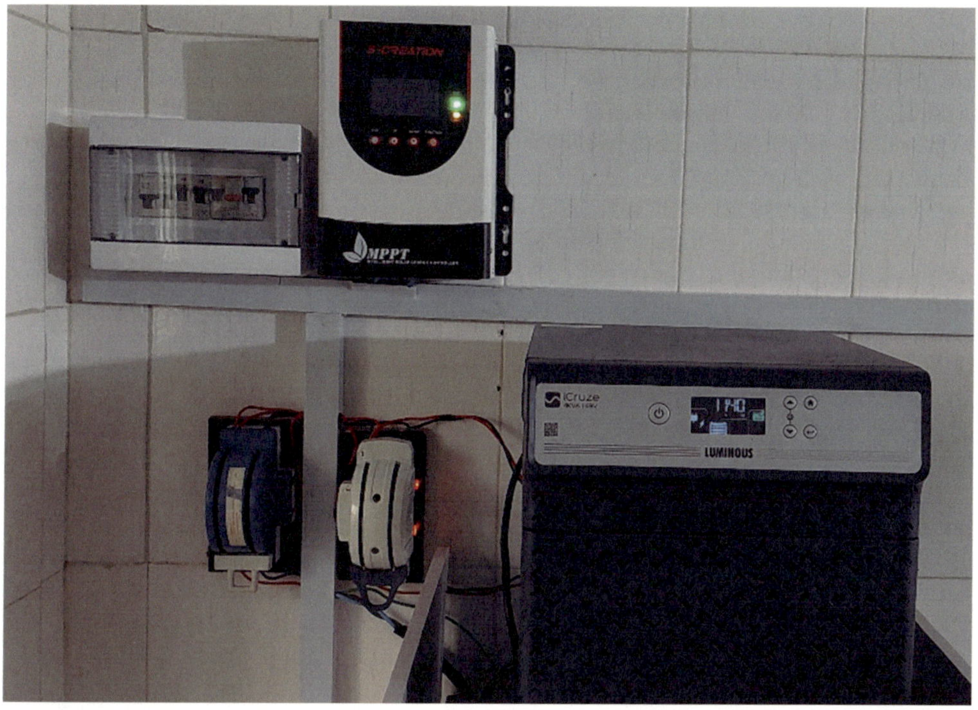

Figure 2.
The solar-subpower unit anchoring the RespSS at UBTH.

when extremely necessary, as the neonates recovered more quickly on their preserved organic surfactant through the pulmonary physiologic warmth promptly delivered by the PoliteHeart CPAP's inspiratory gas.

3. Case 1: First twins after five consecutive neonatal losses – RespSS success in a baby with congenital heart disease

3.1 Background and clinical presentation

Baby O.J. (Twin 1), a male infant, was delivered at 25 weeks and 3 days' gestation via spontaneous vaginal delivery (SVD), weighing 880 g. He was the product of a long-awaited twin pregnancy following five previous unsuccessful pregnancies. On admission at two hours of life, he presented with signs of respiratory distress and was found to have subcostal recession (SCR). A further clinical workup revealed the presence of acyanotic congenital heart disease.

The initial diagnosis was extremely low birth weight (ELBW) preterm with RDS, complicated by congenital heart disease – an ominous combination in a resource-limited setting. There was intense panic in the air as these seemed to replicate the pattern of the previous losses. Little hope was, nevertheless, anchored on the fact that a different intervention technique was about to be used to confront the present case.

3.2 Intervention within the RespSS

The neonate was sub-admitted to the RespSS, and interventions using the PoliteHeart CPAP machine and its oxygen supply systems – the PSS – were initiated at two hours of life. The neonate remained in the RespSS corner for a total of 34 days, supported with additional interventions including surfactant administration, caffeine citrate, antibiotics, anti-failure medications, and transfusions. At this early stage of the RespSS application, the SCBU management recommended the compulsory prophylactic administration of pharmaceutical surfactant, contrary to the RespSS suggestive guidelines. The SCBU management issued this order as a cautionary measure while the RespSS characterization was being established. Therefore, beyond the initial two cases, this cautionary measure was declared needless and was discontinued, only to be used on a patient-specific basis when clinically necessary.

3.3 Outcome and follow-up

By day 33, the baby began experiencing recurrent apnoeic episodes, requiring escalation of care. He was referred to a tertiary facility for mechanical ventilation. Despite the congenital anomaly and a prolonged course on the RespSS systems, the infant was eventually discharged home after 70 days of admission – a significant triumph considering his birth weight and comorbidities. However, it must be noted that this case was one of the initial cases when our practitioners were still carefully learning the applications of the RespSS devices, especially the PoliteHeart CPAP machine.

Hence, the management of this case took a prolonged time to achieve success, as this could have easily been achieved in less than half of this duration, given the current knowledge level at the UBTH RespSS.

3.4 Why this case is compelling

This was the first successful use of the RespSS devices in a neonate with congenital heart disease at UBTH. The emotional background – a mother's first living child after five failed births – adds weight to the clinical triumph. It highlights both the resilience of the neonate and the life-saving capacity of the RespSS gadgets in high-risk, complex conditions. Hence, the successful outcome of this case was a boost to the hopes that would soon become our culture at the substation.

4. Case 2: The second miracle – twin brother overcomes extreme prematurity in the RespSS

4.1 Background and clinical presentation

Born just minutes after his twin brother, Baby O.J. (Twin 2) was delivered at 25 weeks and 3 days via SVD, weighing 860 g. Like his sibling, he was admitted at two hours of life with respiratory distress and was later diagnosed with an atrial septal defect (ASD).

4.2 Intervention in the RespSS

He was promptly initiated on the RespSS devices and managed to achieve total breathing independence in 35 days and was subsequently sub-discharged to the regular care of the open SCBU. The neonate finally received SCBU discharge and went home with the parents after a grand total of 50 days. The additional treatment included antibiotics, caffeine citrate, and surfactant therapy, which had been administered prior to RespSS sub-admission.

4.3 Outcome and follow-up

By its operational guideline, the patient's oxygen requirements, as monitored via the PoliteHeart CPAP system's inbuilt pulse oximeter, would signal when to commence the gradual reduction process of the fraction of inspired oxygen. This process, called the 'algorithmic FiO_2 reduction towards atmospheric (AFRETA)', was signalled for engagement by the fifth day on the device. The algorithmized oxygen dependence reduction, based on the neonate's instantaneous saturation (SpO_2), continued until he was successfully weaned off the PoliteHeart CPAP's PEEP. He achieved independent breathing after 35 days of support in the RespSS corner and was successively sub-discharged back to the open SCBU for continuing care. He remained stable, continued to gain weight, and was finally discharged home weighing 1,650 g. Follow-up confirmed adequate weight gain and no immediate complications.

4.4 Why this case is compelling

This baby represents a second miracle in a high-risk twin pregnancy after multiple previous losses. His steady response in the RespSS, despite his ELBW and cardiac anomaly, underscores the role of efficient early respiratory support in reducing neonatal mortality in preterm infants [7].

5. Case 3: When CPAP applications fail – a rapid turnaround in a 34-week preterm

5.1 Background and clinical presentation

Baby O., a 34-week male preterm infant weighing 2.4 kg, was delivered via caesarean section (C-section) and admitted to the SCBU at 4 hours of life with severe respiratory distress. His oxygen saturation level (SpO_2) remained between 55% and 65% despite treatment using a bubble CPAP (BCPAP) apparatus (Vayu Bubble CPAP System, Vayu Global Health Innovations, 22 Welgate Road Medford, MA 0,2155). The Silverman–Anderson Score for the neonate was 5, indicating moderate distress.

5.2 Intervention with RespSS

Owing to the failure of the BCPAP to improve oxygenation, the patient was transferred and sub-admitted to the RespSS, and PoliteHeart CPAP intervention was initiated. He was managed with antibiotics and caffeine citrate. By day 3, the clinical situation had remarkably improved, and independent breathing was fully achieved. The neonate was monitored for another 24 hours.

5.3 Outcome and follow-up

The baby was fully weaned off the RespSS activities on day 4 and sub-discharged back to the SCBU open hall, having spent a total of only five days in respiratory support. He remained stable and was eventually discharged in good health.

5.4 Why this case is compelling

This case demonstrates the life-saving potential of the RespSS systems and their algorithmized protocols when a regular BCPAP fails, offering a rapid and effective alternative in preterm neonatal care in a resource-limited low- and middle-income country (LMIC) centre such as the SCBU of UBTH, Benin-city. The baby's mother, a parity-5 (Para 5) woman with only one living child before this, adds a layer of emotional significance to this successful outcome.

6. Case 4: *In Vitro* Fertilization victory – RespSS support for twins born after 16 years of waiting

6.1 Background and clinical presentation

Baby O.B. (Twin 1), a male infant born at 26 weeks' gestation via C-section, weighed 1.08 kg at birth. The baby was the product of an *in vitro* fertilization (IVF)-assisted twin gestation, conceived after 16 years of secondary infertility. He was admitted at one hour of life with mild SCR and was diagnosed with preterm very-low birth weight (PTVLBW) and RDS.

6.2 Intervention in the RespSS

Prior to the referral and admission of the neonate for support, the RespSS staff team members had achieved a good level of understanding of how the PoliteHeart CPAP machine could assist in ensuring the preservation of the neonate's organic surfactant via a prompt physiological thermoneutral state for the lungs. This rare skill eliminated the need for prophylactic top-up or replacement with pharmaceutical surfactant. This move resulted in quicker recovery, improved success rates, and completely removed the huge costs associated with surfactant administration. Therefore, for Baby O.B., the RespSS intervention was started within the first hour of life and continued for only six days before the neonate gained breathing independence. The infant also received antibiotics and caffeine citrate.

6.3 Outcome and follow-up

The recovery was strangely swift compared to what our SCBU was used to. Hence, by day 2, the neonates had demonstrated signs of significant respiratory distress reduction. He was eventually weaned off the PoliteHeart CPAP in the RespSS on day 5 and sub-discharged in readiness for the SCBU's full discharge back to his home at a weight of 1.7 kg.

6.4 Why this case is compelling

This baby was part of an IVF twin gestation following decades of infertility. His survival marks not just a clinical victory but a deeply personal one for the parents. The RespSS special devices, especially the PoliteHeart CPAP, played a pivotal role in securing this long-awaited change of situation for the family. It was one of the major eye-openers for our RespSS team, practically demonstrating that sustained and adequate pulmonary warming encourages the natural production of organic surfactant in the lungs for efficient respiration. Using this capability, the PoliteHeart CPAP ensured adequate pulmonary warming, preventing the reduction of organic surfactant production and minimizing pulmonary vasoconstriction, as has been indicated in the literature [6].

7. Case 5: Second chance at fatherhood – RespSS saves IVF twin from respiratory distress

7.1 Background and clinical presentation

The second twin, Baby O.B. (Twin 2), was delivered at 26 weeks via C-section, weighing 1.1 kg. He presented with SCR and had an SpO_2 of 80%. He was diagnosed with PTVLBW and RDS.

7.2 Intervention in the RespSS

The infant was admitted to the RespSS and was commenced on the PoliteHeart CPAP treatment within the first hour. The machine support continued for six days, during which the baby also received antibiotics and caffeine citrate treatment.

7.3 Outcome and follow-up

The patient maintained a stable condition, and by day 3, the signs of an improving situation became evident based on the physiological need to commence the gradual lowering of the fraction of inspired oxygen. The AFRETA – algorithmic protocol was strictly followed, and the baby was weaned off the PoliteHeart CPAP system by day 5. He was eventually discharged at 1.7 kg, healthy and stable.

7.4 Why this case is compelling

This baby was one of two precious lives born after 16 years of infertility through IVF. The RespSS systems ensured that both twins survived and went home – an outcome filled with hope, especially for the couples who had a prolonged, difficult reproductive history. This raised the confidence of practice in our wider SCBU, as the unit had little hope of successfully saving these babies.

8. Case 6: Against the odds – a 1.07 kg preterm beats recurrent apnoea in the RespSS

8.1 Background and clinical presentation

Baby O.S., a female preterm infant born at 28 weeks and 6 days via SVD, weighed 1.07 kg. She was admitted at 36 hours of life with severe respiratory distress, recurrent apnoea, and desaturation (SpO_2 74%) despite early onset of intervention in SCBU using regular techniques with the conventional BCPAP.

8.2 Intervention with RESPSS

Owing to the imminent danger of losing the child as desaturation continued while on the BCPAP, the patient was referred to the RespSS. The PoliteHeart CPAP intervention was initiated. She received antibiotics and caffeine citrate. Respiratory stability and physiological oxygen saturation were achieved within a few hours, and by the second day, the neonate showed marked clinical improvement as the need to commence the algorithmic lowering of oxygen fraction became evident. Hence, AFRETA was initiated. This process went smoothly and was completed quicker than expected within the following 12 hours of the algorithm.

8.3 Outcome and follow-up

The patient achieved the last step of the algorithm, which is the round of gradual removal of PEEP without oxygen supplementation, on the third day. The infant was able to achieve unassisted breathing on the same day and was weaned off the PoliteHeart CPAP and sub-discharged back to the SCBU. She remained stable and was finally discharged home at a weight of 1.68 kg.

8.4 Why this case is compelling

This baby overcame multiple challenges: low birth weight, severe apnoea, and failure of standard CPAP. The RespSS gadgets, especially the PoliteHeart CPAP system, provided a successful rescue strategy. The infant's mother's obstetric history – Para 7 with only two living children – added to the urgency and emotion of this clinical success.

9. Case 7: The first full-term baby admitted to the RespSS – surviving severe birth asphyxia

9.1 Background and clinical presentation

Baby O.F., a term male neonate weighing 2.8 kg, was delivered via emergency C-section for antepartum haemorrhage due to placenta previa. He was unconscious at birth, with an SpO_2 of 65%, and diagnosed with severe birth asphyxia and hypoxic-ischemic encephalopathy (HIE stage 3).

9.2 Intervention with RespSS

The patient was referred to the RespSS after two hours of life following the failure of our regular BCPAP intervention. The neonate was also treated with anticonvulsants and antibiotics. The PoliteHeart CPAP device promptly stabilized the neonate and helped to maintain his breathing while recovering from the deep distress. The usual AFRETA – algorithmized gradual reduction of the fraction of inspired oxygen commenced and progressed seamlessly until total freedom from supplementary oxygen.

9.3 Outcome and follow-up

The baby improved gradually and steadily, and by day 7, his respiratory distress had resolved. He was weaned off the PoliteHeart CPAP and sub-discharged from the RespSS by day 8. He was finally discharged home from the SCBU on oral phenobarbital. He remained stable on follow-up.

9.4 Why this case is compelling

This was the first term baby in UBTH who was managed in the RespSS. Success was achieved in as little as 8 days, which demonstrated that the PoliteHeart CPAP's excellent respiratory efficiency could also be extended to support full-term infants with severe perinatal asphyxia, especially when regular BCPAP proves ineffective.

10. Case 8: Tiny breech survivor – 870 g baby gains independent breathing with RespSS

10.1 Background and clinical presentation

Baby J.B., a 26-week-and-5-day preterm female, was delivered via assisted breech extraction, weighing only 870 g. She was diagnosed with perinatal asphyxia and extreme prematurity.

10.2 Intervention with RespSS

The PoliteHeart CPAP device was initiated at four hours of life and maintained for five days. She received caffeine citrate and antibiotics. The application's three-stage routine was carefully followed as: (1) deliver fully assisted breathing until stability and constant oxygen saturation have been consolidated and the patient shows signs of progress, (2) initiate the algorithmized gradual reduction of the fraction of inspired oxygen until the neonate could be sustained without any supplementary oxygen but on atmospheric air with a PEEP, and (3) initiate and complete the round of algorithmized gradual withdrawal of the PEEP until the neonate could independently sustain its breathing without the water pressure.

10.3 Outcome and follow-up

The infant's condition began to improve after day 2, following which the algorithm for the gradual withdrawal of oxygen was commenced on the PoliteHeart

CPAP. The process towards breathing independence was successfully completed on the fourth day, and the neonate was promptly sub-discharged to the open SCBU. However, the final discharge date and follow-up from the SCBU were not properly documented for inclusion in this report. Nonetheless, the early success of this infant during the RespSS sub-admission was remarkable.

10.4 Why this case is compelling

This case illustrates the PoliteHeart CPAP's capacity to stabilize extremely premature infants delivered via difficult breech extraction, a feat that was habitually rare in our regular experience. It showcases how the RespSS's devices, and particularly the PoliteHeart CPAP, can serve as a critical bridge in the absence of invasive ventilation.

11. Case 9: Triplet with no mother – the RespSS steps in after tragedy strikes

11.1 Background and clinical presentation

Baby O.B. (Triplet-3), a male triplet born at 30 weeks' gestation via emergency C-section for severe pre-eclampsia, weighed 1.23 kg. He was admitted within the first hour with apnoea, hypothermia, and an SpO_2 of 46%. He was diagnosed with RDS and disseminated intravascular coagulation (DIC).

11.2 Intervention with the RespSS

The neonate was given caffeine citrate and antibiotics upon admission to the RespSS. The PoliteHeart CPAP intervention was commenced immediately with close observations.

11.3 Outcome and follow-up

The neonate's vital signs were well maintained, and adequate respiration was sustained by the devices at the RespSS. The signs of consolidated improvement, stability, and readiness for the algorithmized gradual lowering of the FiO_2 were evident by day 4. This was promptly commenced and smoothly progressed to the point of weaning-off from the PoliteHeart CPAP by day 5. The neonate was finally discharged, having improved in weight to 1.7 kg. However, his mother, a 50-year-old IVF patient, passed away from complications one week after delivery.

11.4 Why this case is compelling

The emotional weight of maternal loss following a rare IVF-conceived triplet pregnancy makes this story particularly striking. The RespSS initiative, with all the innovative technologies that drive it, has helped this neonate survive against both clinical and emotional odds.

12. Case 10: Twin sisters' fight – one baby's journey after losing her mother

12.1 Background and clinical presentation

Baby O.B. (Triplet-1), a female triplet born at 30 weeks via emergency C-section, weighed 1.26 kg. She was admitted with apnoea and SpO_2 of 54% and was diagnosed with severe RDS.

12.2 Intervention in the RespSS

Respiratory support via the PoliteHeart CPAP was initiated within the first hour after birth. The neonate was administered caffeine citrate and antibiotics. The formal protocols of the RespSS were carefully followed as the patient was patiently monitored until consolidated stability and readiness for gradual FiO_2 lowering. The AFRETA process was smoothly completed on the fifth day of life when the neonate gained full independent breathing and was subsequently sub-discharged.

12.3 Outcome and follow-up

The patient's initial condition improved, and she was promptly sub-discharged in a stable, independent-breathing condition to continue with other aspects of the specialist care in the SCBU. This was a success for the RespSS, as its mission was successfully achieved. However, the neonate later passed away after developing complications of cellulitis and aspiration in the wider SCBU.

12.4 Why this case is compelling

The baby's initial survival with the RespSS interventions was a clinical win. However, her later death speaks of the ongoing vulnerabilities of preterm infants, even after respiratory stabilization and the independent-breathing feat. Her mother's death cast a sombre shadow over her short life, making this one of the most emotionally intense cases in the series.

13. Summary

The 10 cases presented illustrate the spectrum of very ill neonates who habitually stand little or no chance of survival in LMIC centres, such as in Nigeria, mostly due to inefficient intervention techniques against neonatal respiratory and thermoneutral failures. The RespSS at UBTH was installed as a special intervention technique that could help improve the survival rate of these neonates. Neonatal respiratory disorder has a high incidence rate among our neonatal population, and this facilitates a swift progression to mortality. The RespSS is an initiative aimed at creating a sub-specialty unit within the existing SCBU or the neonatal intensive care unit (NICU) to aid such high-risk neonates and protect them from a rapid decline to mortality due to respiratory distress. Neonates who are already admitted for neonatal care in the SCBU but further present with severe respiratory distress are transferred to the RespSS for specialist respiratory care. They are later sub-discharged back to the main SCBU after gaining breathing independence at the RespSS.

The cases presented here, among 34 others, included extremely preterm infants weighing less than 900 g, very-low-birth-weight twins and triplets (some conceived through IVF after long-standing infertility), term infants with severe birth asphyxia, and neonates with congenital heart disease. These are categories of neonatal cases that would not normally survive prior to the installation of the RespSS. In many instances involving the current cases, conventional respiratory support devices in the main SCBU had failed before the infants were stabilized after referral to the RespSS.

Most of the infants achieved independent breathing within a few days of initiation on the RespSS's PoliteHeart CPAP machine, with subsequent sub-discharge back to the main SCBU for ongoing care. Overall, these cases highlight the capacity of locally innovated respiratory support systems and initiatives to provide effective and sustainable rescue in high-risk neonatal conditions that would otherwise carry a poor prognosis in low-resource settings.

14. Conclusions

The 10 case reports showcased in this chapter may almost sound alike in nature, but each of these represents the nearly impossible cases that drive Nigeria's ever-high neonatal mortality rate, which has defied the efforts of over 4,000 articles from Nigerians in 32 years of scholarly literature [7]. We found it profound and intriguing that a homemade initiative and intervention, such as Hippolite's RespSS, could enter the arena and, with just a stroke, deliver the high-level neonatal survival and confidence that represents our current practice in the UBTH substation.

The combination of all the RespSS devices is streamlined to proactively remove all the well-known bottlenecks of maintaining uninterrupted, successful neonatal care in the Nigerian context. The PoliteHeart CPAP machine delivered an efficient technique for ensuring adequate breathing and ensuring that our neonates were free from complications related to pharmaceutical surfactant requirements. The PSS ensured that we had an adequate oxygen supply and distribution simultaneously to all our patients, as it expanded our one-source input to four independently controlled patient outlets. The RespSS's solar-driven subpower station and power-banking-system ensured that the RespSS, and hence the patients therein, never faced the well-known regular outages or epileptic power supply issues in Nigeria. The interactive AFRETA – algorithm for gradually lowering the fraction of inspired oxygen was the golden technique that eclipsed the whole experience, demonstrating that any neonate could survive if the carer knew what to do.

Having delivered a 100% (34/34) success rate out of all the 34 SCBU referrals received in the 12 months of operating the RespSS initiative at the UBTH, we can confidently affirm that these 34 potential early mortalities were not saved by chance. We have repeatedly succeeded with this initiative and can conclude that LMICs, such as Nigeria, could possess what it takes to stop the regular drivers of high neonatal mortalities without much cost. All the clinical and nursing team members of RespSS at UBTH Nigeria confidently regard this intervention as 'the gating of the superhighway to early neonatal mortality in our setting'.

14.1 Recommendation

The RespSS technologies are sustainable, as they have been maintained over the past 12 months. The system designer is a Nigerian, and the device manufacturing, installations, training, and maintenance were carried out in Nigeria by Nigerians. Therefore, wider usage and application, in our opinion and experience, will guarantee the saving of many dying babies in Nigeria and other LMICs. A scaleup of our UBTH experience across the nation could bring Nigeria's high neonatal mortality narrative to an end. The assistance of philanthropists and healthcare donor institutions is recommended to help fund our hospitals to acquire this technology and save lives.

Acknowledgements

We wish to thank the other members of our RespSS team at the University of Benin Teaching Hospital for their hard work. We appreciate the support from the Chief Medical Director of UBTH and the Nigeria Liquefied Natural Gas (NLNG) Limited, who funded the project. We appreciate all the technical support from the field engineers of Neonatal Concerns for Africa—a collaboration with Imperial College London—who installed the devices and delivered the initial training we needed.

Author details

Ebenovbe Idemudia[1], Ann Brai[1] and Hippolite O. Amadi[2*]

1 Department of Paediatrics, University of Benin Teaching Hospital, Benin-city, Nigeria

2 Department of Bioengineering, Imperial College London, London, United Kingdom

*Address all correspondence to: h.amadi@imperial.ac.uk

References

[1] WHO. 2024. Fact Sheet, Newborn Mortality. World Health Organisation Newsroom [Internet]. Available from: https://www.who.int/news-room/fact-sheets/detail/newborn-mortality [Accessed: 2025-September-11]

[2] Amadi HO, Abubakar AL. Neonatal respiratory support substations within Nigerian special care baby units: A noteworthy initiative. Journal of Pediatrics and Neonatal Care. 2025;**15** (1):47–50. DOI: 10.15406/jpnc.2025.15.00582

[3] Amadi HO, Okonkwo IR, Abioye IO, Abubakar AL, Olateju EK, Adesina CT, Umar S, Eziechila BC. A new low-cost commercial bubble CPAP (bCPAP) machine compared with a traditional bCPAP device in Nigeria. Paediatrics and International Child Health. 2019; **39**(3):184–192. DOI: 10.1080/20469047.2019.1598125

[4] Amadi HO. The Politeoxygen Splitter System (PSS) – A frugal LMIC oxygen delivery technology that expands the utility by up to 700%. Journal of Paediatrics and Neonatal Care. 2023;**13**(2):75–80. https://medcraveonline.com/JPNC/JPNC-13-00495.pdf

[5] Amadi HO, Abubakar AL. LMIC facility-lighting limitation in Nigeria fully resolved by a novel frugal Polite-light-bank technology. Global Journal of Medical Research GJMR-K. 2023;**23**(3). Version 1.0. https://globaljournals.org/GJMR_Volume23/1-LMIC-Facility-Lighting-Limitation-in-Nigeria.pdf

[6] Carns J, Kawaza K, Quinn MK, Miao Y, Guerra R, Molyneux E, Oden M, Richards-Kortum R. Impact of hypothermia on implementation of CPAP for neonatal respiratory distress syndrome in a low-resource setting. Public Library of Science One. 2018;**13** (3):e0194144. DOI: 10.1371/journal.pone.0194144

[7] Amadi HO, Abioye IO, Ugbolue UC, Ekpenyong R-D, Ekwem NF, Nwaneri OJ, Dike C. The case of the neonate vs. LMIC medical academia—a jury-style systematic review of 32 years of literature without significant mortality reduction. Frontiers in Pediatrics. 2024;**12**:1413113. DOI: 10.3389/fped.2024.1413113

Section 3

Drug-resistant Epilepsy

Chapter 4

Treating Drug-Resistant Epilepsy: Describing the Phase 1 and Phase 2 Presurgical Evaluations for Definitive Management

Derryl Joseph Miller, Taylor N. Parrish, Sofia A. Giannini and Trisha Lea Miller

Abstract

Following the diagnosis of epilepsy, two-thirds of patients are made seizure-free by the prescription and titration of appropriate antiseizure medications (ASMs) at therapeutic doses. For the one-third of patients who have drug-resistant epilepsy (DRE), treatment with ASMs alone is unlikely to achieve seizure freedom, with odds of about 1 in 20. For this reason, it is critical that providers diagnosing DRE, defined as the failure of two appropriately chosen ASMs at high therapeutic doses for efficacy, execute a phase 1 presurgical evaluation at their center or refer patients to a National Association of Epilepsy Centers (NAEC) Level 4 facility as soon as possible. For those patients who are candidates for resective or ablative surgery for the potential cure of their epilepsy, surgery may immediately proceed from the phase 1 evaluation in cases of high concordance of data, or a phase 2 evaluation can be conducted to map eloquent cortices or further refine the surgical hypothesis for targeted intervention. For those patients who are determined to be poor candidates for resection or ablation surgery, palliative surgery such as neuromodulation or disconnection can be considered, along with further ASM trials and the ketogenic diet. This chapter is a comprehensive review and summary of the literature for the provider caring for patients with DRE requiring maximal medical, dietary, and surgical care.

Keywords: epilepsy, seizures, antiseizure medications, ketogenic diet, phase 1 evaluation, phase 2 evaluation, epilepsy surgery, neuromodulation

1. Introduction

Patients with epilepsy suffer from a predilection to have seizures, with the risk of recurrence of seizures being 60% or greater [1, 2]. The patient with epilepsy has three major treatment options, including antiseizure medications (ASMs), dietary therapies, and epilepsy surgeries with curative and palliative intent [2]. As most patients with epilepsy respond to ASMs and become completely seizure-free, ASMs are generally selected as the first-line treatment to utilize unless dietary therapy or surgery is clearly indicated for their specific pathology (e.g., SLC2A1 gene mutation or high-grade central nervous system tumor requiring resection). ASMs rendering a patient seizure-free are generally continued for a time until the patient's risk of recurrence of seizures is estimated to be low [2]. Reestimation of the risk of recurrence of seizures is possible after a prolonged period of seizure freedom, which is generally two or more years, when ASMs may be cautiously weaned if head imaging and the electroencephalogram (EEG) show a low risk of recurrence of seizures [2]. For those patients who do not become seizure-free with medications alone, the diagnosis of drug-resistant epilepsy (DRE) is made, and additional treatment options are considered, which will be detailed in this Chapter [2].

2. Diagnosing drug-resistant epilepsy

Epilepsy is diagnosed when a patient has a seizure and a high risk of recurrence of seizures (≥60%), estimated by the number of previous seizures, the EEG, structural imaging of the brain with magnetic resonance imaging (MRI) and computed tomography (CT), and genetic studies such as chromosome microarray or next-generation sequencing, including gene panels, whole exome sequencing, or whole genome sequencing [1–3]. Treatment of patients with epilepsy using ASMs has been previously described, and ASMs are generally the first selected treatment for seizures if diagnostics do not suggest that a surgical or dietary/supplement approach is superior [2–7]. For one-third of patients with epilepsy, seizure freedom is not achieved after trialing two appropriately chosen ASMs, at which point a diagnosis of DRE is appropriate, despite having over 30 ASMs available for titration [2, 8–10].

Patients with DRE have an increased risk of sudden unexplained death in epilepsy (SUDEP) compared to patients with medication-responsive epilepsy, especially if they have frequent seizures or nocturnal generalized tonic-clonic seizures [11, 12]. For patients with DRE, SUDEP risk reduction requires control of seizures through titration of ASMs, the ketogenic diet, and epilepsy surgery [12].

3. Assessment of the cause of drug-resistant epilepsy

When DRE is diagnosed, a thorough search for its cause is necessary. DRE is a heterogeneous disease, including genetic causes of seizures, acquired epilepsy from previous brain lesions, and inflammatory/metabolic causes, which are often intractable to ASMs [2, 3, 13, 14]. While epilepsy syndromes may aid in the initial identification of seizures and initiation of appropriate ASMs, epilepsy etiologies remain heterogeneous within discrete syndromes, necessitating an etiology-level diagnosis for tailored treatment [15]. Furthermore, nonepileptic diagnoses mimic DRE, such as attention deficit hyperactivity disorder, autism spectrum disorder, and psychogenic nonepileptic seizures (PNES), which do not respond to ASMs due to not being epileptic seizures [16–19]. Video EEG is the gold standard to spell capture events and differentiate between nonepileptic mimics and DRE [2, 8, 19]. DRE requires a significant workup, including next-generation sequencing, metabolic testing (including lactate, pyruvate, ammonia, serum amino acids, urine organic acids, mucopolysaccharides from urine, carnitine and acylcarnitine profile analysis, branch chain amino acids, and very long chain fatty acids), detailed neuroimaging and magnetic resonance spectroscopy (MRS), and serum and cerebrospinal fluid studies for autoimmune encephalitis acquired via lumbar puncture [2, 14].

Once epilepsy etiology is known, tailored therapies such as additional vitamins, dietary modification, or ASM choice can be directed for efficacy even before DRE is diagnosed. However, patients with DRE may also have highly efficacious therapies made available through etiologic diagnosis rather than continuing to treat them with only a syndromic diagnosis [2–6, 20–24]. Epilepsy syndromes can still be useful for the early diagnosis and early empiric choice of ASMs while diagnostics are performed to clarify the epilepsy etiology [25].

4. Phase 1: Presurgical evaluation

Once DRE is diagnosed, surgical treatment options that are efficacious can and should be determined by completing a phase 1 presurgical evaluation [2]. The phase 1 presurgical evaluation is noninvasive and involves overlapping data to build concordance and certainty in the suggested surgical approaches to treat the patient [2, 26]. Concordance is required for successful epilepsy surgery, as the goal of efficacious epilepsy surgery is to remove or destroy the epileptogenic zone, which is the smallest region of the brain that, if removed or destroyed, would resolve DRE completely [26, 27]. Delineating the epileptogenic zone is challenging, as there is no perfect measurement to define its complete extent [2, 26, 27]. Noninvasive testing can present a hypothesis of the location and extent of the epileptogenic zone by measuring other parameters [26, 27]. To hypothesize the location of the epileptogenic zone, we measure the irritative zone, the functional deficit zone, the symptomatogenic zone, the seizure onset zone, and the lesional zone [2, 26].

The irritative zone is detected interictally by measuring the regions of the brain from which interictal epileptiform abnormalities are observed, often through a brief scalp EEG test, acquiring an interictal 18F-Fluorodeoxyglucose positron emission tomography computed tomography (FDG-PET/CT), which detects regions of the brain that poorly metabolize glucose between seizures, interictal Technetium-99 m single-photon emission computed tomography (SPECT), and magnetoencephalography (MEG) [2, 26, 28, 29].

The functional deficit zone refers to the regions of the brain that function poorly between and after seizures, which are best detected through mental status testing with neuropsychological testing [30]. Serial neuropsychological testing is also performed preoperatively to detect the progression of disease and postoperatively to assess the effects of epilepsy surgery [31, 32]. Epilepsy surgery can also result in some cognitive improvements in patients who experience successful destruction of the epileptogenic zone [32]. Lastly, the functional deficit zone may also include motor, sensory, visual, language, and other focal neurologic deficits, which can be detected by the astute provider during physical examination [33, 34].

The symptomatogenic zone is determined by history. The patient describes their perception of the seizures, caregivers describe what they witness, and videos are analyzed for clinical cues to localize the seizures [35]. Seizure semiologies can vary significantly across the frontal, temporal, parietal, occipital, and insular lobes, and semiologic analysis can further subcategorize the seizure symptomatogenic zone within these lobes [35, 36]. One very interesting sign is ictal pouting, also known as the "chapeau de gendarme" sign, referring to the bicorn hat of the French police, which localizes well to the anterior cingulate gyrus of the frontal lobe [37].

The seizure onset zone is measured using both electric and magnetic fields, which are orthogonal to each other [38]. The postsynaptic potentials produced by ions in the brain traveling through channels to depolarize and hyperpolarize neurons are measured by placing electrodes on the scalp utilizing the international 10–20 system [39, 40]. The ictal pattern on scalp EEG can often provide helpful lateralizing and localizing data for seizures, but the spatial resolution of these abnormalities within the brain is often poor due to the attenuation of signals through healthy brain parenchyma, the skull, and the scalp [41]. MEG detects magnetic fields around the head, which are generated by orthogonal electric fields, and magnetic fields are not attenuated by the layers of overlying brain, skull, and scalp [42]. By solving the inverse problem, magnetic field data can produce high spatial resolution of electric fields within the brain, both for measuring interictal and ictal foci [43]. There is also an ictal injection of the Technetium-99 m SPECT, which can be utilized to make a subtraction scan called subtraction ictal SPECT coregistered to MRI (SISCOM) when an interictal SPECT is subtracted from an ictal SPECT [28, 44].

Lesions in the brain are highly suggestive of involvement in the epileptogenic zone and may have a high overlap with the epileptogenic zone if they are highly epileptogenic lesions [45]. Examples of highly epileptogenic lesions include mesial temporal sclerosis, cortical dysplasia (polymicrogyria, pachygyria, periventricular nodular heterotopia, lissencephaly, schizencephaly), epileptogenic tumors such as dysembryoplastic neuroepithelial tumor, and other disorders of the gray matter such as ischemic or hemorrhagic stroke with encephalomalacia, postsurgical lesions, and inflammatory lesions [2, 45]. Detecting these lesions is best accomplished with highly sensitive imaging, such as MRI of the brain with higher-strength magnets of 3–7 tesla [46]. These high-quality MRI images have high voxel density to improve the detection of small gray matter lesions predisposing the patient to seizures [46].

Following the collection of adequate data for a noninvasive phase 1 presurgical evaluation, patients are discussed at our center in a multidisciplinary epilepsy surgery committee, with input from epileptologists, neurosurgeons, clinical neurophysiologists, neuropsychologists, and neuroradiologists, to establish the degree of confidence in the concordance of the data [2]. Our procedure for the diagnosis of epilepsy, acquisition of phase 1 presurgical data, discussion in the presurgical conference, and surgical determination is shown in **Figure 1**.

The committee determines whether surgery candidacy is already clear due to high concordance of data, whether additional phase 1 testing is needed to formulate a more precise hypothesis of the extent of the epileptogenic zone, or whether invasive phase 2 monitoring is needed either to increase the precision of the surgical intervention or for cortical mapping of suspected eloquent cortices [47–54]. With discordance in phase 1 presurgical data and the presence of gene mutations portending the risk of progressive or diffuse disease, the epilepsy surgery committee may decide that the patient is not a good candidate for resection or ablation surgery but may benefit from palliative surgery, additional ASMs, or the ketogenic diet [2, 3]. Given the complexity of the phase 1 presurgical evaluation process, the durations of evaluation are variable, and analyses of the factors that delay or expedite testing for patients with DRE to determine surgical candidacy have been published [55].

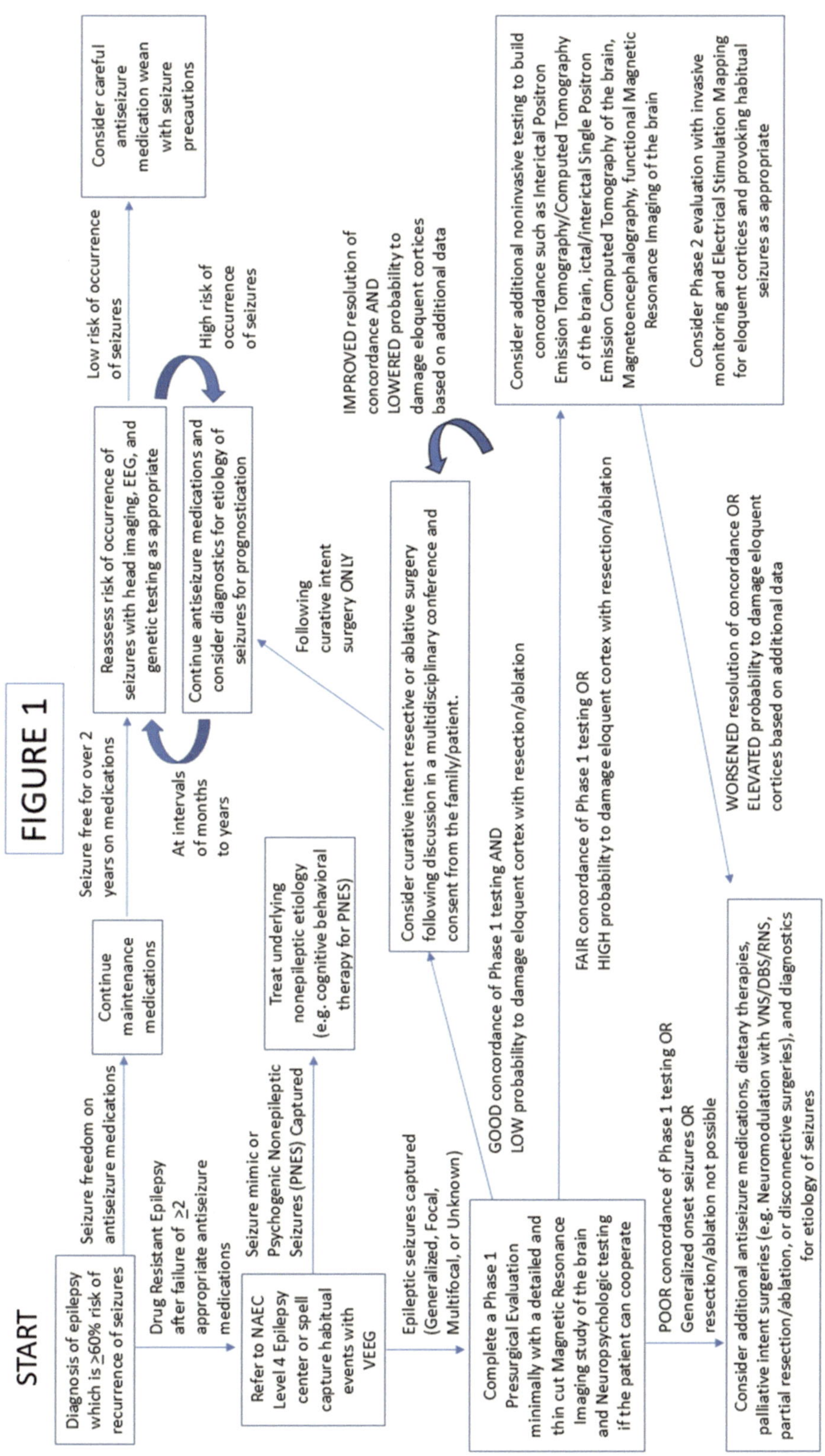

Figure 1.
Procedure for the diagnosis of epilepsy and guiding patients toward, through, and away from the presurgical evaluation based on their response to treatment.

4.1 Noninvasive mapping techniques

Functional MRI of the brain, MEG, and Wada testing are all utilized to lateralize the patient's language and motor cortices to prevent injury to these eloquent regions when planning epilepsy surgery. This evaluation is especially important in patients who are left-handed or who have had injury to the suspected dominant hemisphere from stroke or other previous pathology, as language lateralization is not clearly delineated in these groups. The goal of phase 1 presurgical evaluation is definitive epilepsy surgery with ablation or resection, which remains the most efficacious intervention, or lateralization or localization of the seizure focus, prompting additional studies or a phase 2 presurgical evaluation.

5. Phase 2: Surgical evaluation

If lateralization is achieved but localization is unclear after a comprehensive phase 1 presurgical evaluation, phase 2 presurgical evaluation improves precision with surgically implanted grid, strip, depth, or stereoelectroencephalography (sEEG) electrodes. The placement of electrodes is guided by the epileptologist and neurosurgeon to more accurately localize the patient's seizure onset zone for definitive surgical treatment [26]. At times during the phase 1 or phase 2 evaluation, the patient is determined not to be a candidate for resection or ablation surgery due to the epileptogenic zone being multifocal, generalized, or involving eloquent cortices [18, 26]. Rather than performing disabling resective or ablative surgery in these cases, palliative surgery, additional ASM trials, and dietary management with the ketogenic diet are possible [40, 43]. Electrical stimulation mapping (ESM) during phase 2 evaluation is also performed by the epileptologist by delivering small shocks to each implanted contact to determine the location of eloquent cortices at the bedside, an additional advantage of phase 2 evaluation [26].

5.1 Direct electrical stimulation mapping technique and parameters

Exact parameters of ESM for eloquent cortices and habitual seizure provocation are not firmly established [47–49]. ASMs can decrease the risks of after-discharges (ADs) and seizures. A retrospective pediatric ESM study reported seizures in 23% of 40 patients premedicated with fosphenytoin 10–20mgPE/kg IV, compared to 43% in 82 nonpremedicated patients [50].

ESM broadly has two goals: 1) mapping eloquent cortices and 2) eliciting habitual seizures if none are captured spontaneously [51]. At our center, high-frequency stimulation is used for mapping eloquent cortices, and low-frequency stimulation is used for seizure provocation, as shown in **Table 1**.

Setting	Functional mapping	Seizure provocation
Frequency (Hz)	50	1
Pulse duration (msec)	0.2–0.3	0.1–0.5
Duration (seconds)	1–5	1–30

Table 1.
Parameters for seizure provocation and functional mapping, respectively.

While grids and strips provide better density and delineation of ESM, sEEG allows for bilateral and multilobar sampling of the brain, and both methods are used in ESM [52]. Grids or strips at our center have circular electrodes with a diameter of 2.4 mm, which are 10 mm apart. sEEG uses deep electrodes, which are 0.8–0.86 mm in diameter, inserted into the brain with 5–18 cylindrical contacts depending on the electrode length of 2–2.29 mm, which are 1.5–10 mm apart (DIXIT®, ADTech®) [53, 54]. sEEG is used to map the functions and connections of fiber bundles [56]. Charge density delivered to the brain determines the upper limit of safe ESM, and the literature/manufacturer suggests a maximal charge density of 30–50 μC/cm^2 [57].

$$\textbf{Charge Density}\ (\boldsymbol{\mu}\mathbf{C/cm^2}) = [\textbf{Stimulation Intensity}\ (\mathbf{mA})]*[\textbf{Pulse Duration}\ (\mathbf{msec})]/\textbf{Electrode Surface Area}\ (\mathbf{cm^2})$$

For grids/strip electrodes, the surface area (SA) is 0.0452 cm^2 (0.12 cm$\cdot$0.12 cm$\cdot\pi$), so for a maximal charge density of 30–50 μC/cm^2, the maximal stimulation intensity and pulse duration are shown in **Table 2**.

For sEEG electrodes, SA is constant at 0.081 cm^2 per the manufacturer, so for a maximal charge density of 30–50 μC/cm^2, the maximal stimulation intensity and pulse duration are shown in **Table 3.**

Stimulation at each target site should begin at a low current intensity and be titrated. The train duration depends on the task. Shorter durations are commonly used for motor mapping, while longer durations are preferred for language mapping to allow sufficient time for the patient to undergo multiple trials of the language task. We stimulate suspected eloquent cortices first and seizure generators last. This is to optimize confidence in mapping eloquent cortices before inducing seizures, which cause functional deficits. For sEEG, stimulating deep electrodes first reduces the chance of

Pulse duration (msec)	Max stimulation (mA) for 30 μC/cm^2 limit	Max stimulation (mA) for 50 μC/cm^2 limit
0.5	2	4
0.4	3	5
0.3	4	7
0.2	6	11
0.1	13	22

Table 2.
Maximal safe grid/strip electrode pulse duration and stimulation intensity.

Pulse duration (msec)	Max stimulation (mA) for 30 μC/cm^2 limit	Max stimulation (mA) for 50 μC/cm^2 limit
0.5	4	8
0.4	6	10
0.3	8	13
0.2	12	20
0.1	24	40

Table 3.
Maximal safe sEEG electrode pulse duration and stimulation intensity.

stimulating the dura mater, which can be painful, and triggering seizures or ADs early, which compromises confidence ESM foruredloquent cortices. We increase stimulation by 1–2 mA increments until one of the following is observed: 1) a clinical effect, 2) the maximum stimulation intensity is reached for safety, or 3) ADs or seizures are noted. If ADs or seizures are noted, it is advised to consider pausing the ESM if there are concerns that this activity may impact the clinical assessment of eloquent cortices that remain to be mapped. If eloquent cortices are adequately mapped, stimulation for seizures may proceed after addressing ADs or seizures that are not habitual.

If ADs are noted but no clinical effects are seen, consider the following: higher frequency (100 Hz vs. 50 Hz) and longer pulse width (1 msec vs. 0.2 msec) are more likely to cause ADs. The occurrence of ADs can compromise the safety and neurophysiologic validity of ESM, as an associated functional response being attributable to stimulation or ADs becomes difficult to distinguish. In the case of ADs remote from the site of stimulation, localization of any observed behavioral response to the stimulated cortical site versus the region showing ADs remains unclear. If ADs/seizures are seen, it is advisable to repeat the stimulation after an interval of 15–30 minutes, during which time testing can be conducted on other electrode contacts. When retesting contacts where previous stimulations had induced ADs, we begin stimulation at 1–5 mA below the previous ADs threshold.

Eloquent cortices are often well-preserved, but their exact location can be difficult to determine in patients with a previous brain injury. The expected locations of eloquent cortices are listed in **Table 4**.

ESM for the motor cortex involves stimulating and observing for movement contralaterally from the electrode. If ESM induces mild dysesthesia, repeating stimulation at 0.5–1 mA higher intensity may determine whether a motor response can be induced. If a positive motor response is induced, the dysesthesia was from subliminal motor activation of muscle fibers, while the induction of pain in the craniofacial region suggests cranial nerves or dural structures were stimulated [49]. ESM for the language cortex is not standard, as there is no consensus on a unified clinical language testing protocol, but we stimulate while administering multiple language tasks specifically oriented to the targeted language site [53]. Broca's area function is impacted when patient tasks for naming difficulties are impaired, followed by reading difficulties and, less likely, automatic speech impairments. Wernicke's area function is impacted when the patient has naming difficulties and reading aloud

Eloquent cortex	Expected location
Primary motor cortex	Frontal lobe in the contralateral precentral gyrus
Primary sensory cortex	Parietal lobe in the contralateral postcentral gyrus
Primary visual cortex	Occipital lobe near the contralateral medial calcarine sulcus
Primary auditory cortex	Temporal lobe in the Sylvian fissure at the transverse gyrus of Heschl, represented bilaterally
Primary motor speech cortex	Dominant frontal lobe in the opercular structures at the pars opercularis and pars triangularis
Primary sensory speech cortex	Dominant temporal lobe in the posterior aspect of the superior temporal gyrus

Table 4.
Eloquent cortices and their expected anatomic locations in most patients. Damage to eloquent cortices results in major neurological deficits, so localization of these cortices by ESM can prevent disabling surgical lesions.

difficulties, with less repetition impairment. Arcuate fasciculus function is impacted when the patient is unable to complete repetition tasks. An alternative language mapping approach with intracranial recordings consists of observing for high-frequency activity on the background tracing with language tasks such as visual or auditory naming. Intracranial recordings may also show an auditory-language-related gamma-increase, which can provide additional information useful to localize eloquent language areas [53]. ESM for the visual cortices is achieved when the patient reports contralateral visual phenomena during stimulation. ESM for the sensory cortices is accomplished when the patient tells us if they experience tactile sensation changes during contralateral stimulation. ESM for memory involves sending stimulation and then showing the patient a picture to recall, removing the picture before stimulation is complete, and requesting the patient to remember the object that was shown. ESM of the insula for eloquent function is generally not necessary, as the insula is rarely an eloquent cortical structure, but ESM of the insula may result in phenomena that are part of the habitual seizure [58].

6. Epilepsy surgery

Following the acquisition of high concordance of data suggesting highly effective and safe surgical techniques for the treatment of DRE, epilepsy surgery may be performed [2, 59]. Epilepsy surgery broadly refers to surgical techniques aimed at reducing seizures, which can involve cerebral surgery with resection, ablation, disconnection, or neuromodulation, or peripheral neuromodulation for the reduction of seizures [2, 59]. Epilepsy surgery has two major goals of treatment: curative intent and palliative intent [2, 59]. Curative intent surgeries have a high probability of achieving seizure freedom, while palliative surgeries result in seizure reduction without the expectation of seizure freedom [2, 59]. These surgical techniques, while having acute risks, also have high efficacy for the resolution and reduction of seizures relative to medical management alone, which has already failed patients with DRE [2, 59, 60]. Curative surgeries generally involve resection or ablation of a portion of the brain hypothesized to be the epileptogenic zone, while palliative surgery involves disrupting the network with ablation, resection, disconnection, or neuromodulation [2, 59]. The risks and benefits of epilepsy surgery should favor benefit to the patient, but curative surgeries may appropriately have greater postoperative risk than palliative surgeries to balance this risk.

6.1 Minimally invasive laser interstitial thermal therapy

When epilepsy surgery is indicated for lesions that are small or for nonlesional epilepsy localized with sEEG, minimally invasive surgical techniques with magnetic resonance guided laser interstitial thermal therapy (MRgLITT) can be performed [59]. MRgLITT does not require a craniotomy and utilizes avascular trajectories with preoperative MRI to implant lasers, which can use thermal ablation to damage approximately a 4 mm cylindrical trajectory. This trajectory can be placed with submillimetric precision into deep structures and small lesions (e.g., hypothalamic hamartoma, periventricular nodular heterotopia, cortical tubers) [59]. The thermal damage of MRgLITT is monitored actively utilizing magnetic resonance thermography and the Arrhenius equation, which is an integral of damage over time calculated with temperature and constants related to protein denaturation [59–61]. MRgLITT has also been used for disconnection procedures such as corpus callosotomy, and MRgLITT has successfully lateralized an ictal pattern in both adults and children previously in those with poorly lateralized ictal onset during phase 2 monitoring procedures [59, 62, 63]. By lateralizing the ictal onset with MRgLITT, additional surgery can resolve epilepsy, even in those with poorly lateralized intracranial EEG monitoring [62, 63].

6.2 Intraoperative neuromonitoring during resective surgery

While minimally invasive surgery has many practical applications, as previously discussed, large regions, large lesions, or areas proximal to eloquent cortices may require open resective surgery [2, 59, 64]. Open resection is performed with stereotactic precision to determine the location of the craniotomy to expose the surgical field, and once the entry trajectory is exposed, intraoperative neuromonitoring is performed to facilitate safe surgery, reduce disability postoperatively, and improve the precision and efficacy of surgery [64–70]. After exposing the brain, eloquent surface cortices are established by stimulating the median nerve at the wrist while placing a grid or strip of electrodes perpendicularly to the hypothesized hand knob in the precentral gyrus and the postcentral gyrus to identify the cortical surface "phase reversal," which is the cortical somatosensory evoked potential – a negative waveform at the postcentral gyrus and a precentral positive potential detected in adjacent electrodes [68, 69]. Following the positive identification of these cortices, baseline direct cortical motor evoked potentials are achieved by applying stimulation to the precentral gyrus medially and laterally while recording with electromyography distally [69]. When applying current to the cortex of the brain, electrocorticography (ECoG) is performed on the surface of the brain away from the stimulation site to detect provoked seizures and spontaneous discharges and seizures to guide resection through the irritative and seizure onset zones [64, 65, 66, 67, 68, 69]. Periodic monitoring of motor evoked potentials and somatosensory evoked potentials can detect changes in waveform amplitude and complexity, which indicate lesions in these critical pathways, while subcortical mapping with current applied to resective tools detects eloquent white matter tracts to avoid injury to these critical structures [64, 69, 70]. Even if a patient receiving epilepsy surgery had prophylactic ASMs, the epileptologist may detect seizures while monitoring ECoG during resection, which can be treated by applying iced sterile solutions (e.g., normal saline or lactated ringers) to the brain, followed by intravenous treatment with in line benzodiazepines or propofol if total intravenous anesthesia is utilized, and loads of ASMs such as levetiracetam 15–60 mg/kg intravenously [71–73]. When appropriately utilized, intraoperative neuromonitoring has lowered rates of postoperative motor, sensory, and language deficits in both spine and brain surgeries [74–77].

The largest resection and disconnection procedures, which have curative intent, include hemispherectomy and functional hemispherotomy [78]. In patients with hemispheric disease, hemispherectomy and functional hemispherotomy both have high rates of cure, about 77%, with a reduction of seizures for most other patients who do not achieve a cure [78]. Because hemispherectomy and functional hemispherotomy necessitate disruption/resection of eloquent cortices, postoperative deficits are expected, including contralateral hemiparesis, contralateral homonymous hemianopsia, contralateral sensory changes, potential language deficits, and neurocognitive changes. However, earlier age of surgery allows plasticity of the other hemisphere to recover lost functions, improving outcomes [78–80].

6.3 Curative-intent epilepsy surgeries and outcomes

Resective and ablative surgery carry differing rates of highly favorable Engel 1 outcomes, and rates of seizure freedom are estimated based on cohort studies in **Table 5** [81–91].

Engel 1 outcomes are also improving over time due to improvements in surgical techniques, presurgical precision, and advances in phase 2 neuromonitoring [92]. There is some attrition of Engel 1 surgical outcomes with prolonged follow-up of months to years in the literature, suggesting surgical outcomes are best shortly after surgery but can also be sustained in the majority of cases [85, 86, 91]

6.4 Palliative intent epilepsy surgeries/neuromodulation techniques

Palliative intent epilepsy surgery is intended to reduce seizures without the expectation of seizure freedom [2]. There are currently multiple devices available for neuromodulating seizures, which stimulate peripherally or centrally and are open-loop or closed-loop [2, 59]. Neuromodulation successfully reduces seizures and SUDEP, though it has only a low chance of cure [2, 59, 93–95]. Other palliative intent surgeries, such as partial resection, corpus callosotomy, and multiple subpial transection, can be performed to reduce seizures for the purposes of improving quality of life and titrating off ASMs, but palliative surgeries are of lower efficacy than curative intent resection and ablation. Palliative surgery should be offered to patients in whom curative surgery is unlikely to result in seizure freedom or carries a high risk for postoperative disability [2].

7. Ketogenic diet therapy: History and utilization

Ketogenic diet therapy (KDT) has been a treatment for epilepsy since biblical times and has been utilized more frequently since 1921 [96]. The Charlie

Lesion/location and procedure	Engel 1 surgical outcome
Rasmussen's encephalitis with hemispherectomy or functional hemispherotomy	75–85%
Hypothalamic hamartoma with laser interstitial thermal therapy	67–77%
Mesial temporal sclerosis with anterior temporal lobectomy	60–80%
Mesial temporal sclerosis with laser interstitial thermal therapy	52–79%
Lesion-negative mesial temporal seizures with resection or laser interstitial thermal therapy	43–67%
Extratemporal lesional epilepsy with resection	62–83%
Extratemporal lesional epilepsy with laser interstitial thermal therapy	41–59%
Extratemporal nonlesional epilepsy with phase 2 monitoring	12.5–38%

Table 5.
Postoperative rates of Engel 1 surgical patients (considered a cured state) who may succeed in weaning from ASMs for many common surgeries.

Foundation (1994) and Matthew's Friends (2004) became the two support groups that helped medical centers all over the world establish and create programs for KDT [97, 98]. Within the last 20 years, KDT has been more widely used and researched and remains an established treatment option for children and adults with DRE [99–102]. This chapter highlights the process by which ketogenic dietitians (KDs) and epileptologists/neurologists from Riley Hospital for Children start and maintain both pediatric and adult patients on KDT in accordance with previous protocols [98]. These processes and recommendations are evidence-based and developed with input from different medical centers as well as consensus guidelines and research [96–102]. When patients have DRE and are not candidates for definitive surgery, or if the family prefers additional nonsurgical and nonmedical therapies for epilepsy, the low glycemic index (LGI) diet, modified Atkins diet (MAD), and ketogenic diet can be utilized for both generalized and focal onset seizures [96–102]. The international recommendations for offering KDT include patients with DRE who are not surgical candidates [100].

KDT is a high-fat, adequate-protein, and minimal-carbohydrate diet that promotes the use of fat as the primary fuel for the brain [98]. When carbohydrates and protein are restricted, the mitochondrial beta-oxidation of fat occurs in the liver and produces large quantities of acetoacetate and beta-hydroxybutyrate, which are used as an energy source and are measured in the serum and urine [98, 100]. The exact mechanism of KDT for treating epilepsy is not fully understood [98]. A ketogenic diet ratio is the comparison of grams of fat to grams of carbohydrate and protein combined (fat: carbohydrate + protein) [97]. The efficacy of KDT is that about 50% of patients experience a > 50% reduction in seizures, and 10–15% will become seizure-free [98]. The 2018 Consensus Guidelines for the management of children on KDT outlined syndromes and conditions for which KDT has been consistently beneficial, moderately beneficial, or contraindicated, with such conditions listed in **Table 6** [98].

7.1 Ketogenic diet therapy: Initial evaluation/assessment

The neurologist/epileptologist will send appropriate patients to the KD if they feel the patients would be the best candidates for initiating KDT. The patient is required to obtain baseline fasting blood work to assess their current nutritional status and to ensure there is nothing that would contraindicate a high-fat diet [98]. This blood work includes CBC with differential, CMP, phosphorus, magnesium, lipid panel, vitamin D, free and total carnitine analysis, prealbumin, lactate, ammonia, uric acid, zinc, selenium, plasma amino acid, acylcarnitine analysis, ferritin, urine amino acid, and urine organic acid screen [98]. ASM levels or other tests may be added by the physician to assess a baseline prior to the initiation of KDT. Once these labs are processed, the neurologist will review and approve the patient as clinically safe to start diet therapy. If there is concern with the results of the blood work, the physician may choose to refer the patient to another provider for further work-up, and KDT will not be initiated. If the blood work comes back within normal limits, the neurologist/epileptologist will give the KD the approval to continue. Additional vitamin/mineral supplementation or free water will be recommended at this point to correct any baseline deficiencies or other abnormal nutrition-related values [98].

Epilepsy syndromes > 50% responsive to KDT	Epilepsy syndromes moderately responsive to KDT	Contraindications to KDT
Angelman syndrome	CDKL5 encephalopathy	Primary carnitine deficiency
Doose syndrome (epilepsy with myoclonic-atonic seizures)	Cortical malformation disorders (holoprosencephaly, lissencephaly, pachygyria, polymicrogyria, schizencephaly)	Carnitine palmitoyltransferase 1 or 2 deficiency
Dravet syndrome (SCN1A)	Developmental epileptic encephalopathy with spike-wave activation in sleep (DEE/SWAS)	Carnitine translocase deficiency
Febrile infection related epilepsy syndromes	Glycogenosis type V	Beta-oxidation defects (short-chain, medium-chain, or long-chain acyl dehydrogenase deficiency)
Infantile spasms	Idiopathic generalized epilepsies (childhood absence epilepsy, juvenile absence epilepsy, and juvenile myoclonic epilepsy)	Pyruvate carboxylase deficiency
Mitochondrial disorder of complex 1	Lafora body disease	Porphyria
Ohtahara syndrome	Landau-Kleffner syndrome/acquired epileptic aphasia	Recurrent pancreatitis or kidney stones on the diet
Pyruvate dehydrogenase deficiency	Lennox-Gastaut syndrome	Use of propofol for the treatment of seizures
Super-refractory status eplepticus	Rett syndrome	Highly efficacious epilepsy surgery exists for the patient
Tuberous sclerosis	Subacute sclerosing panencephalitis	Weight loss despite maximal intervention

Table 6.
Epilepsy syndromes with high and moderate responses to KDT, as well as contraindications to KDT.

7.2 Antiseizure medications and the ketogenic diet

Any and all medications will be converted to the lowest carbohydrate-containing form, most of which require switching from liquid to tablet, capsule, or sprinkle forms, as many liquid medications have added sugar [98]. If medications cannot be converted into tablet/capsule/sprinkle form due to dosing restrictions or issues with administration, the amount of carbohydrate from the liquid medication will be noted and calculated into the diet ratio or feeding plan. It is important to note that carbohydrates from the tablet or capsule form of medications are still calculated into the diet ratio, as many medically complex patients are on several medications, which may add additional grams of carbohydrates. The recommendation at our center is to have no more than 1 g of carbohydrates from all medications.

At our center, the KD conducts a phone or in-person consultation to assess baseline nutrition history and evaluation prior to starting KDT. The KD fills out an *Intake Form* to document the history. This intake form includes information such as parent contact information, baseline height or length/weight/body mass index or weight-for-length, pertinent medical history and diagnosis, ASMs and dosages, seizure patterns, bowel habits, activity/developmental level, food allergies and intolerances, swallowing or Video Feeding Swallow Study (VFSS) results, therapies, seizure goals, and diet expectations. For patients who have gastrostomy or jejunostomy tubes, an enteral feeding history is also obtained (e.g., type of feeding tube, enteral formula, feeding schedule, additional free water, previous enteral formulas trialed, home care, or nursing company).

After completing the KD assessment, intake form, and reviewing KDT basics with the family, the KD sends a follow-up email with more information. This email includes additional websites and resources that may be useful for families to learn more about KDT. Several handouts are attached to this email: *Clinic Handout FAQ, Charlie Foundation FAQ, Charlie Foundation Statistics, General Information about KDT at Riley Hospital for Children, Ketogenic Diet Fact Sheet, and compiled Ketogenic Diet Resources.* If the patient is enterally fed, a list of formula options is provided for parents to conduct their own research and notify the KD of which formula they would like to choose for their child; otherwise, the KD will select the most appropriate option based on their medical history [98]. The KD encourages families to review all of the resources and handouts and then follow up with the KD with any further questions [98]. Lastly, the next steps for KDT initiation are listed at the end of the email to the family. If the family decides not to continue with the process, the KD will notify the medical team and will not proceed with further steps. Additionally, if the KD notes there are barriers to education or concerns with the current nutrition history, KDT initiation will be discontinued.

7.3 Initiating the ketogenic diet

For orally or enterally fed patients, there are several options for commercial ketogenic ready-to-feed formulas available in different ketogenic diet ratios – 2.43:1, 2.5:1, 3:1, 4:1; however, these formulas can be customized to meet the patients' nutritional needs and specific diet ratios with modulars and other food ingredients [98]. There are plant-based ketogenic formula options for patients who may have allergies or intolerance to milk, some with added medium chain triglyceride (MCT) oil, different flavors (vanilla/chocolate/unflavored), and an organic whole food plant-based blended product. The KD can also curate a home tube feeding blend that can be customized to the patients' cultural foods or allow them to personalize and create more variety in the patient's diet.

For those patients who eat food orally, before KDT can be initiated, two to three days' worth of food records are requested to assess current intake, feeding schedule, and typical foods and recipes the child or adult is already eating. Once the food records are returned, KD will utilize Cronometer and/or KetoDietCalculator™ to assess current intake. KD will assess for oral supplements, as there are documented benefits to utilizing a keto oral supplement to help meet fat and fluid goals. For those patients who have a G-tube, this can also be beneficial to use for medication administration, additional fluids, liquid fat, and/or formula supplementation [103].

If the initial evaluation and assessment are complete, and the family is interested in continuing the process, the KD will schedule another phone call, telehealth session, or in-person visit with the family. If the patient is non-English speaking, an in-person appointment with an in-person interpreter is preferred. At Riley Hospital, the KD initiates KDT in the ambulatory care setting. Inpatient diet initiation for enterally fed patients is only considered if the patient is in the neonatal intensive care unit (NICU), is in status epilepticus, or is medically complex.

The KD will meet with the family to review some documents that are utilized while the patient is on KDT. An enteral feeding plan and an over-the-counter medication guide are sent via email or presented to the family in person to review.

When creating the enteral feeding plan, KDT is started at a 1:1 diet ratio, or roughly half of the patient's previous enteral formula and the new ketogenic enteral formula [98, 100]. The nutrient composition for every patient is entered into KetoDietCalculator™ to ensure that the patient is meeting their electrolyte, vitamin, and mineral needs [103]. Any additional supplements are added to personalize the plan to the patient's needs. Common household items, such as table salt, baking soda, lite salt, or salt substitute, are added to ensure electrolyte needs are met. KDT has a diuretic effect, which can lead to a loss of sodium, potassium, and chloride [98]. As for vitamin/mineral needs, and depending on the formula, a nutrient-dense multivitamin powder can also be added to the tube feeding regimen. Chewable or tablet multivitamins can also be utilized but are not as nutritionally complete. Depending on the baseline labs, iron, cholecalciferol (vitamin D3), and levocarnitine may be supplemented to correct deficiencies [98]. After the patient is on this first step for at least 7–10 days, they are instructed to acquire blood work. A basic metabolic panel (BMP) and beta-hydroxybutyrate level are obtained to assess electrolyte and blood ketone levels. The KD will review these labs and make adjustments to the feeding plan if necessary. Then the KD will send the new plan and increase the ratio by 0.5–1 at a time. Blood work is completed after every step of the diet. In younger patients, weekly weight checks at a local pediatrician's office are recommended to ensure adequate calories are being given for optimal growth. After one month postdiet initiation, a free and total carnitine analysis is obtained to ensure that the patient has not developed a deficiency. The goal diet ratio is set with beta-hydroxybutyrate levels, with a maximum of 5–6 mmol/L, or seizure control [98].

For a patient who eats orally, KD meets with the family to review a KDT packet containing in-depth information about carbohydrates, protein, fat, sick day guidelines, fat sources, snack and meal examples, prepackaged and specific "keto" brands available, and kitchen staples. KD will also review the patient's feeding plan, go over KetoDietCalculator™, and assist in creating and reviewing keto meals and snacks [103]. After this initial appointment, the family will start with one keto meal per day, focusing on three to five recipes per meal. After about five to seven days, the family will advance to two meals per day and aim to focus on three to five recipes for this next meal. Once halfway to full KDT initiation, the patient will undergo lab tests to check beta-hydroxybutyrate and BMP to assess tolerance and level of ketosis. Contingent on normal limits, the patient will continue to include additional meals and snacks every three to five days until all meals and snacks are keto meals. Once all meals and snacks are keto, the patient will undergo lab tests again after maintaining the goal for five to seven days, including carnitine levels.

At Riley Hospital, there are lab order sets that the KD can recommend. A "Ketogenic Diet 3 Month Lab Order set" contains beta-hydroxybutyrate, CBC with Differential, CMP, Phosphorus, and Magnesium. A "Ketogenic Diet 6 Month Lab Order set" contains CMP, magnesium, phosphorus, lipid panel, uric acid, beta-hydroxybutyrate, prealbumin, free and total carnitine analysis, zinc, selenium, CBC with differential, and ferritin. A "Ketogenic Diet 12 Month Lab Order set" is a six month set with a vitamin D level added. Other labs may be ordered, such as additional vitamin and mineral levels, inflammatory markers, and ASM levels.

Once the patient is stable on KDT, a neurology/KD appointment is scheduled every three months, especially during the first year on KDT. Appointments can then be spaced out to every six months if the patient remains stable after one year. At the three-month mark of starting KDT, the efficacy of KDT and how it has impacted the patient's seizure control will be analyzed. If families do not note a change in seizure control, and the diet has been fully optimized, KDT will be discontinued at this time. Research has shown that patients do not need to be weaned off the diet in a stepwise fashion and can return to their normal formula. However, tolerance is best if their previous formula is reintroduced similarly to the first step of diet initiation. Blood work is also obtained one to two weeks prior to every neurology/KD appointment to assess electrolyte and vitamin levels, ensuring that no dietary changes need to be made and that there are no nutritional deficiencies or concerns. During these follow-up appointments, if the diet can be adjusted over ASMs, this is preferred. Bowel habits, blood or urine ketone levels, energy levels, nutrition-focused physical exams (NFPE), and anthropometrics are also assessed at these appointments. ASMs and diet ratio changes will not be made concurrently, which can help to discern if KDT has an impact on seizure control. Between clinic visits, the KD team remains available via phone or telehealth visits, assisting the patient and family with KDT.

Riley Hospital for Children has unique support for patients who eat orally. There are quarterly virtual support groups that discuss something educational related to KDT, provide an opportunity for discussion among all participants, as well as feature a new recipe demonstration. There is a quarterly newsletter that is sent out the month after the support group. This newsletter includes a recap from the support group, a local grocery haul, tips from a fellow keto parent, a new recipe, as well as product highlights and any upcoming networking and educational opportunities. Four times a year, a holiday newsletter is sent out (Easter, Fall, Thanksgiving, and Christmas) to help families normalize these holidays by recommending nonfood ideas, as well as seasonal recipes that are all appropriate while on the KDT. Lastly, there is an in-person support group that takes place at Riley and includes a keto-friendly pitch-in, activities, door prizes, as well as participation in the Purple Pumpkin Project.

7.4 Acute side effects of the ketogenic diet

Several acute side effects of KDT are discussed with the family prior to KDT [98]. These side effects are closely monitored and managed throughout the entire process. Constipation is one of the most common side effects that patients experience on KDT [98]. The use of polyethylene glycol powder, sennosides (tea or tablets), saline enemas, magnesium citrate (vitamin), or high-fat foods like avocado and MCT oil can be effective in managing constipation. Our patients are advised to aim for daily or every-other-day bowel movements to prevent intolerance or other unwanted side effects.

Elevated blood lipids can occur when KDT is initiated but will typically normalize within 6 months of being on KDT. If lipid levels continue to remain elevated, carnitine therapy, omega-3 supplementation, replacing fats with MCT oil, reducing the KDT ratio, limiting cholesterol-rich foods, sunflower lecithin, and increasing plant fiber may be initiated. While children on KDT do not develop atherosclerotic disease, arterial stiffness is observed with chronic treatment [100].

Metabolic acidosis from low serum bicarbonate is another common acute side effect associated with the use of KDT. Higher beta-hydroxybutyrate levels correlate with lower blood bicarbonate levels [98]. Adding a bicarbonate supplement of around 2–3 milliequivalents per kilogram, dosed twice per day, as well as increasing free water in the feeding plan, has been effective for treatment [98]. Decreasing or weaning certain ASMs, such as topiramate, zonisamide, and acetazolamide, which are carbonic anhydrase inhibitors (CA–I), should be considered when initiating KDT, as CA–I can also cause metabolic acidosis, which can prevent optimization of KDT [98].

Fatigue can occur due to the body's change in metabolic processes. As carbohydrates are decreased, there is a fluid and electrolyte shift in the body, due to carbohydrates holding onto water where electrolytes are present in the body. This is commonly referred to as the "keto flu" but can be avoided by slowly initiating KDT in a stepwise fashion, as well as by meeting fluid and electrolyte needs [98]. Additionally, free and total carnitine analysis is consistently monitored to ensure that these levels are optimal for patients on KDT, as a deficiency may cause fatigue.

Growth and development may be impacted on KDT [97, 98]. Excessive calorie intake can cause rapid weight gain and decrease levels of ketosis, whereas inadequate calorie intake can result in poor growth and insufficient ketosis [97, 98]. Calorie and protein needs are continually adjusted during KDT to ensure adequate weight and height growth occur. Nutritional deficiencies can occur in patients on KDT. The smaller volume of food that the patient is consuming due to a high diet ratio, along with severely limiting food groups, can lead to nutritional deficits. Obtaining blood work and frequent NFPE can diagnose and treat these deficiencies. Some patients can also struggle with formula intolerance, especially those who are medically complex with frequent viral or respiratory illnesses, or those who struggle with the management of constipation [98]. KDT can exacerbate these medical complications but can be managed by diluting regular Pedialyte with water (considered half-strength Pedialyte) for one to two days to help symptoms resolve. Half-strength feeds, calculated by the KD, are resumed after the half-strength Pedialyte to help with tolerance. Stepwise introduction of formula reduces dehydration by providing electrolytes, fluids, and some carbohydrates to help prevent excessive ketosis [98]. Depending on the severity of the illness or intolerance, KD and the physician may recommend an emergency department evaluation if the patient may need intravenous fluids. Dehydration occurs more frequently and rapidly when on KDT due to the lower amount of carbohydrates in the body that retain water [98]. BMP and beta-hydroxybutyrate are assessed; based upon those results, KD may recommend dextrose 2.5% normal saline intravenous hydration if ketosis is excessive (>6 mmol/L) for a certain number of hours until ketosis is back within the usual goal range [98]. Fluids and sodium bicarbonate may help with metabolic acidosis or if patients are *nil per os* for a procedure or surgery.

7.5 Long-term use of the ketogenic diet and side effects

Bone health can be a concern in patients on KDT [98]. At Riley Hospital, a dual-energy X-ray absorptiometry (DEXA) scan is completed every two years after KDT initiation. DEXA is available for patients aged ≥5 years. ASMs can also negatively impact bone health, resulting in poor bone mineral density [104]. If the DEXA scan shows osteopenia or osteoporosis, a referral is made to endocrinology for treatment [104]. Nonambulatory patients are at higher risk for poor bone mineral density due to their nonweight-bearing status. Kidney stones are another side effect of KDT [98]. The KD will ensure that free water needs are met at 100–120% of the goal, as well as adding bicarbonates, citrates, and phosphorus to help prevent acidosis and renal stones from forming [98]. The neurologist may again consider weaning off CA–I ASMs, as these can cause acidosis and lead to renal stones [98]. Renal ultrasounds can be obtained every two years after KDT initiation but may be recommended more frequently in patients with a history of kidney stones. Citrates are started if the patient has a history of renal stones prior to or after KDT. The neurologist will also send a referral to urology/nephrology to comanage these patients as indicated [98].

There are many different ways to initiate and adhere to the diet [102]. We have met families who prefer a holistic approach with the highest quality ingredients and supplements, as well as very low-income families with minimal oral variety who rely completely on supplements via prescriptions from KD, achieving success.

7.6 Weaning antiseizure medications after surgery or a ketogenic diet

There is no standard practice for weaning ASMs after epilepsy surgery or KDT with seizure freedom. The current practice is to continue ASMs for months to years and wean one ASM at a time while monitoring for recurrence (**Figure 1**).

8. Conclusions

For the neurologist and epileptologist, many treatments exist for the management of DRE, which is encountered in one-third of patients diagnosed with epilepsy. Treatment options include ASMs, KDT, and curative and palliative intent epilepsy surgeries. The identification of DRE is a critical time for the neurologist to perform a complete phase 1 presurgical evaluation and workup for the etiology of epilepsy while considering the future therapeutic management of any patient not completely seizure-free on the first two appropriately chosen ASMs at high therapeutic doses. The chance of an Engel 1 outcome after curative surgery is higher than with medical and dietary management for patients with DRE, though high-risk surgeries can be avoided with palliative intent surgery or additional dietary or ASM trials. DRE should be managed aggressively to reduce the risk of SUDEP, and patients should be referred to an epilepsy center capable of delivering high-quality dietary and surgical therapies in addition to ASM trials.

Acknowledgments

This chapter was written without funding.

Conflict of interest

There are no conflicts of interest.

Thanks

The authors thank God, their families, their colleagues, and their many teachers for the preparation and inspiration to write this book chapter.

Author details

Derryl Joseph Miller[1*], Taylor N. Parrish[1], Sofia A. Giannini[1] and Trisha Lea Miller[2]

1 Indiana University School of Medicine, Indianapolis, USA

2 Salesforce, Indianapolis, IN, USA

*Address all correspondence to: miller89@iu.edu; dmiller21@iuhealth.org

References

[1] Fisher RS, Acevedo C, Arzimanoglou A, Bogacz A, Cross H, Elger CE, Engel J, Forsgren L, French JA, Glynn M, Hesdorffer DC, Lee BI, Mathern GW, Moshe SL, Perucca E, Scheffer IE, Tomson T, Watanabe M, Wiebe S. ILAE Official Report: A practical clinical definition of epilepsy. Epilepsia. 2014;**55**(4):475–482. DOI: 10.1111/epi.12550

[2] Miller D. Childhood epilepsies and when to refer for epilepsy surgery evaluation. IntechOpen. 2024. DOI: 10.5772/intechopen.1005271

[3] Charouf D, Miller D, Haddad L, White FA, Boustany R-M, Obeid M. High diagnostic yield and clinical utility of next-generation sequencing in children with epilepsy and neurodevelopmental delays: A retrospective study. International Journal of Molecular Sciences. 2024;**25**(17):9645. DOI: 10.3390/ijms25179645

[4] Tang M, Park SH, De Vivo DC, Monani UR. Therapeutic strategies for glucose transporter 1 deficiency syndrome. Annals of Clinical and Translational Neurology. 2019;**6**(9):1923–1932. DOI: 10.1002/acn3.50881

[5] Assi L, Saklawi Y, Karam PE, Obeid M. Treatable genetic metabolic epilepsies. Current Treatment Options in Neurology. 2017;**19**(9):30. DOI: 10.1007/s11940-017-0467-0

[6] Jaafar F, Obeid M. Successful treatment of cerebral folate transporter deficiency with intravenous folinic acid. Pediatric Neurology. 2022;**135**:22–24. DOI: 10.1016/j.pediatrneurol.2022.07.005

[7] Lee JW, Wen PY, Hurwitz S, et al. Morphological characteristics of brain tumors causing seizures. Archives of Neurology. 2010;**67**(3):336–342. DOI: 10.1001/archneurol.2010.2

[8] Kwan P, Arzimanoglou A, Berg AT, Brodie MJ, Hauser WA, Mathern G, Moshe SL, Perucca E, Wiebe S, French J. Definition of drug resistant epilepsy: Consensus proposal by the ad hoc Task FORCE of the ILAE Commission on Therapeutic Strategies. Epilepsia. 2010;**51**(6):1069–1077. DOI: 10.1111/j.1528-1167.2009.02397.x

[9] Moosa ANV. Antiepileptic drug treatment of epilepsy in children. Continuum (Minneap Minn). 2019;**25**(2 Epilepsy):381–407. DOI: 10.1212/CON.0000000000000712

[10] Auvin S, Galanopoulou AS, Moshé SL, Potschka H, Rocha L, Walker MC. Revisiting the concept of drug-resistant epilepsy: A TASK1 report of the ILAE / AES Joint Translational Task Force. Epilepsia. 2023;**64**(11):2891–2908. DOI: 10.1111/epi.17751

[11] Devinsky O, Friedman D, Besag FMC. Nocturnal monitoring in epilepsy: Evidence mounts. Neurology. 2018;**91**(16):731–732. DOI: 10.1212/WNL.0000000000006345

[12] Pathak SJ, Yousaf MIK, Shah VB Sudden unexpected death in epilepsy. [Updated 2022 Dec 19]. In: StatPearls [Internet]. Treasure Island (FL): StatPearls Publishing; 2025. Available from: https://www.ncbi.nlm.nih.gov/books/NBK559104/ [Accessed: 2025-November-13]

[13] Kwan P, Arzimanoglou A, Berg AT, Brodie MJ, Allen Hauser W, Mathern G, Moshé SL, Perucca E, Wiebe S, French J. Definition of drug resistant epilepsy: Consensus proposal by the ad hoc Task Force of the ILAE Commission on Therapeutic Strategies. Epilepsia. 2010;**51**(6):1069–1077. DOI: 10.1111/j.1528-1167.2009.02397.x

[14] Samanta D, Garrity L, Arya R. Refractory and Super-refractory Status Epilepticus. Indian Pediatrics. 2020;**57**(3):239–253. DOI: 10.1007/s13312-020-1759-0

[15] Scheffer IE, Berkovic S, Capovilla G, Connolly MB, French J, Guilhoto L, Hirsch E, Jain S, Mathern GW, Moshé SL, Nordli DR, Perucca E, Tomson T, Wiebe S, Zhang Y-H, Zuberi SM. ILAE classification of the epilepsies: Position paper of the ILAE Commission for Classification and Terminology. Epilepsia. 2017;**58**(4):512–521. DOI: 10.1111/epi.13709

[16] Miller DJ, Komanapalli H, Dunn DW. Comorbidity of attention deficit hyperactivity disorder in a patient with epilepsy: Staring down the challenge of inattention versus nonconvulsive seizures.. Epilepsy & Behavior Reports. 2024;**25**:100651. DOI: 10.1016/j.ebr.2024.100651

[17] Patel H, Blake H, Dunn D. Psychogenic nonepileptic seizures in children and adolescents. Indian Pediatrics. 2021;**58**(3):259–265. DOI: 10.1007/s13312-021-2167-9

[18] Patel H, Dunn DW, Austin JK, Doss JL, LaFrance Jr WC, Plioplys S, Caplan R. Psychogenic nonepileptic seizures (pseudoseizures). Pediatrics In Review. 2011;**32**(6):e66–72. DOI: 10.1542/pir.32-6-e66

[19] McWilliams A, Reilly C, Gupta J, Hadji-Michael M, Srinivasan R, Heyman I. Autism spectrum disorder in children and young people with non-epileptic seizures. Seizure. 2019;**73**:51–55. DOI: 10.1016/j.seizure.2019.10.022

[20] Beniczky S, Trinka E, Wirrell E, Abdulla F, Al Baradie R, Alonso Vanegas M, Auvin S, Singh MB, Blumenfeld H, Bogacz Fressola A, Caraballo R, Carreno M, Cendes F, Charway A, Cook M, Craiu D, Ezeala-adikaibe B, Frauscher B, French J, Gule MV, Higurashi N, Ikeda A, Jansen FE, Jobst B, Kahane P, Kishk N, Khoo CS, Vinayan KP, Lagae L, Lim K-S, Lizcano A, McGonigal A, Perez-gosiengfiao KT, Ryvlin P, Specchio N, Sperling MR, Stefan H, Tatum W, Tripathi M, Yacubian EM, Wiebe S, Wilmshurst J, Zhou D, Cross JH. Updated classification of epileptic seizures: Position paper of the International League Against Epilepsy. Epilepsia. 2025;**66**(6):1804–1823. DOI: 10.1111/epi.18338

[21] Zuberi SM, Wirrell E, Yozawitz E, Wilmshurst JM, Specchio N, Riney K, Pressler R, Auvin S, Samia P, Hirsch E, Galicchio S, Triki C, Snead OC, Wiebe S, Cross JH, Tinuper P, Scheffer IE, Perucca E, Moshé SL, Nabbout R. ILAE classification and definition of epilepsy syndromes with onset in neonates and infants: Position statement by the ILAE Task Force on Nosology and Definitions. Epilepsia. 2022;**63**(6): 1349–1397. DOI: 10.1111/epi.17239

[22] Specchio N, Wirrell EC, Scheffer IE, Nabbout R, Riney K, Samia P, Guerreiro M, Gwer S, Zuberi SM, Wilmshurst JM, Yozawitz E, Pressler R, Hirsch E, Wiebe S, Cross HJ, Perucca E, Moshé SL, Tinuper P, Auvin. International League Against Epilepsy classification and definition of epilepsy syndromes with onset in childhood:

Position paper by the ILAE Task Force on Nosology and Definitions. Epilepsia. 2022;**63**(6):1398–1442. DOI: 10.1111/epi.17241

[23] Riney K, Bogacz A, Somerville E, Hirsch E, Nabbout R, Scheffer IE, Zuberi SM, Alsaadi T, Jain S, French J, Specchio N, Trinka E, Wiebe S, Auvin S, Cabral-lim L, Naidoo A, Perucca E, Moshé SL, Wirrell EC, Tinuper P. International League Against Epilepsy classification and definition of epilepsy syndromes with onset at a variable age: Position statement by the ILAE Task Force on Nosology and Definitions. Epilepsia. 2022;**63**(6):1443–1474. DOI: 10.1111/epi.17240

[24] Hirsch E, French J, Scheffer IE, Bogacz A, Alsaadi T, Sperling MR, Abdulla F, Zuberi SM, Trinka E, Specchio N, Somerville E, Samia P, Riney K, Nabbout R, Jain S, Wilmshurst JM, Auvin S, Wiebe S, Perucca E, Moshé SL, Tinuper P, Wirrell EC. ILAE definition of the Idiopathic Generalized Epilepsy Syndromes: Position statement by the ILAE Task Force on Nosology and Definitions. Epilepsia. 2022;**63**(6):1475–1499. DOI: 10.1111/epi.17236

[25] Wirrell EC, Nabbout R, Scheffer IE, Alsaadi T, Bogacz A, French JA, Hirsch E, Jain S, Kaneko S, Riney K, Samia P, Snead OC, Somerville E, Specchio N, Trinka E, Zuberi SM, Balestrini S, Wiebe S, Cross JH, Perucca E, Moshé SL, Tinuper P. Methodology for classification and definition of epilepsy syndromes with list of syndromes: Report of the ILAE Task Force on Nosology and Definitions. Epilepsia. 2022;**63**(6):1333–1348. DOI: 10.1111/epi.17237

[26] Jehi L. The epileptogenic zone: Concept and definition. Epilepsy Currents. 2018;**18**(1):12–16. DOI: 10.5698/1535-7597.18.1.12

[27] Frauscher B. Localizing the epileptogenic zone. Current Opinion in Neurology. 2020;**33**(2):198–206. DOI: 10.1097/WCO.0000000000000790

[28] Sarikaya I.PET studies in epilepsy. . American Journal of Nuclear Medicine and Molecular Imaging. 2015;**5**(5): 1443–1474

[29] Shiraishi H, Ahlfors SP, Stufflebeam SM, Knake S, Larsson PG, Hämäläinen MS, Takano K, Okajima M, Hatanaka K, Saitoh S, Dale AM, Halgren E. Comparison of three methods for localizing interictal epileptiform discharges with magnetoencephalo graphy. Journal of Clinical Neurophysiology. 2011;**28**(5):431–440. DOI: 10.1097/WNP.0b013e318231c86f

[30] Patrikelis P, Messinis L, Kimiskidis V, Gatzonis S. Neuropsychology of epilepsy surgery and theory-based practice: An opinion review. Arquivos de Neuro-Psiquiatria. 2023;**81**(9):835–843. DOI: 10.1055/s-0043-1770349

[31] Pulsipher DT, Stanford LD. Serial neuropsychological testing before and after hemispherectomy in a child with electrical status epilepticus in slow wave sleep. Epilepsy & Behavior Reports. 2022;**18**:100539. DOI: 10.1016/j.ebr.2022.100539

[32] Sherman EM, Wiebe S, Fay-mcclymont TB, Tellez-Zenteno J, Metcalfe A, Hernandez-Ronquillo L, Hader WJ, Jetté N. Neuropsychological outcomes after epilepsy surgery: Systematic review and pooled estimates.

Epilepsia. 2011;**52**(5):857–869. DOI: 10.1111/j.1528-1167.2011.03022.x

[33] Faust SL, Mattson KS, Felker M, Jordan B, Miller DJ. Focal epileptic encephalopathy with spike-wave activation in sleep: A case report of hemispheric involvement with change in handedness. The Neurodiagnostic Journal. 2025;**65**(2):89–100. DOI: 10.1080/21646821.2025.2484028

[34] Rolak LA, Rutecki P, Ashizawa T, Harati Y. Clinical features of Todd's post-epileptic paralysis. . Journal of Neurology, Neurosurgery & Psychiatry. 1992;**55**(1):63–64. DOI: 10.1136/jnnp.55.1.63

[35] Beniczky S, Tatum WO, Blumenfeld H, Stefan H, Mani J, Maillard L, Fahoum F, Vinayan KP, Mayor LC, Vlachou M, Seeck M, Ryvlin P, Kahane P. Seizure semiology: ILAE glossary of terms and their significance. Epileptic Disorders. 2022;**24**(3):447–495. English. DOI: 10.1684/epd.2022.1430

[36] Bonini F, McGonigal A, Trébuchon A, Gavaret M, Bartolomei F, Giusiano B, Chauvel P. Frontal lobe seizures: From clinical semiology to localization. Epilepsia. 2014;**55**(2):264–277. DOI: 10.1111/epi.12490

[37] Lu H, Zhang W, Liu S, Sun W The chapeau de gendarme sign can be evoked by lateral prefrontal epileptic seizures. Seizure. 2021;**87**:17–20. Epub. DOI: 10.1016/j.seizure.2021.02.024

[38] Stauffer RC. Speculation and Experiment in the Background of Oersted's Discovery of Electromagnetism. Isis. 1957;**48**:33–50

[39] Jasper HH. The 10-20 electrode system of the International Federation. Electroencephalography and Clinical Neurophysiology. 1958;**10**:367–380

[40] Oostenveld R, Praamstra P. The five percent electrode system for high-resolution EEG and ERP measurements. Clinical Neurophysiology. 2001;**112**(4):713–719. DOI: 10.1016/s1388-2457(00)00527-7

[41] Szaflarski JP. The man versus the machine: The machine wins the race to detect the scalp-negative seizures. Epilepsy Currents. 2017;**17**(3):142–143. DOI: 10.5698/1535-7511.17.3.142

[42] Wens V. Exploring the limits of MEG spatial resolution with multipolar expansions. Neuroimage. 2023;**270**:119953. DOI: 10.1016/j.neuroimage.2023.119953

[43] Hämäläinen M, Hari R, Ilmoniemi RJ, Knuutila J, Lounasmaa OV. Magnetoencephalography—theory, instrumentation, and applications to noninvasive studies of the working human brain. Reviews of Modern Physics. 1993;**65**:413–497. DOI: 10.1103/RevModPhys.65.413

[44] Yassin A, El-Salem K, Al-Mistarehi A-H, Momani A, Zein Alaabdin AM, Shah P, Mountz JM, Bagić AI. Use of innovative SPECT techniques in the presurgical evaluation of patients with nonlesional extratemporal drug-resistant epilepsy. Molecular Imaging. 2021;**2021**:6614356. DOI: 10.1155/2021/6614356

[45] Moosa AN, Wyllie E Focal epileptogenic lesions. Handbook of Clinical Neurology. 2013;**111**:493–510. PMID: 23622198. DOI: 10.1016/B978-0-444-52891-9.00053-1

[46] Park JE, Cheong E-N, Jung DE, Shim WH, Lee JS. Utility of 7 tesla

magnetic resonance imaging in patients with epilepsy: A systematic review and meta-analysis. Frontiers in Neurology. 2021;**12**:621936. DOI: 10.3389/fneur.2021.621936

[47] Corley JA, Nazari P, Rossi VJ, Kim NC, Fogg LF, Hoeppner TJ, Stoub TR, Byrne RW. Cortical stimulation parameters for functional mapping. Seizure. 2017;**45**:36–41. DOI: 10.1016/j.seizure.2016.11.015

[48] Jahangiri FR, Dobariya A, Kruse A, Kalyta O, Moorman JD. Mapping of the motor cortex. Cureus. 2020;**12**(9):e10645. DOI: 10.7759/cureus.10645

[49] So EL, Alwaki A. A guide for cortical electrical stimulation mapping. Journal of Clinical Neurophysiology. 2018;**35**(2):98–105. DOI: 10.1097/WNP.0000000000000435

[50] Grande KM, Ihnen SKZ, Arya R. Electrical stimulation mapping of brain function: A comparison of subdural electrodes and stereo-EEG. Frontiers in Human Neuroscience. 2020;**14**. DOI: 10.3389/fnhum.2020.611291

[51] Arya R, Ervin B, Dudley J, Buroker J, Rozhkov L, Scholle C, Horn PS, Vannest J, Byars AW, Leach JL, Mangano FT, Greiner HM, Holland KD, Glauser TA. Electrical stimulation mapping of language with stereo-EEG. Epilepsy & Behavior. 2019;**99**:106395. DOI: 10.1016/j.yebeh.2019.06.038

[52] Cockle E, Rayner G, Malpas C, Alpitsis R, Rheims S, O'brien TJ, Neal A. An international survey of SEEG cortical stimulation practices. Epilepsia Open. 2023;**8**(3):1084–1095. DOI: 10.1002/epi4.12790

[53] Aron O, Jonas J, Colnat-Coulbois S, Maillard L. Language mapping using stereo electroencephalography: A review and expert opinion. Frontiers in Human Neuroscience. 2021;**15**:619521. DOI: 10.3389/fnhum.2021.619521

[54] George DD, Ojemann SG, Drees C, Thompson JA. Stimulation mapping using stereoelectroencephalography: Current and future directions. Frontiers in Neurology. 2020;**11**:320. DOI: 10.3389/fneur.2020.00320

[55] Al-Ramadhani R, Hyslop A, Caraway AR, Novotny EJ, Ostendorf AP, Eschbach KL, Alexander AL, Wong-kisiel LC, Depositario-cabacar DF, Oluigbo CO, Karakas C, Karia SR, Tatachar P, Bolton J, Pichon PD, Shrey DW, Romanowski EF, McNamara NA, Gonzalez-giraldo E, Auguste K, Bernardo D, Singh RK, Javarayee PK, Lin JJ, Coryell JC, Reddy SB, Ganesh A, Ciliberto MA, Samanta D, Arredondo KH, Marashly A, Grinspan ZM, Armstrong D, Abel TJ, Wagner J, Miller DJ, Galan FN, Perry MS. Factors influencing the duration from the initiation of surgical evaluation to final intervention in pediatric epilepsy surgery. Annals of the Child Neurology Society. 2025;**3**:188–200. DOI: 10.1002/cns3.70027

[56] Drane DL, Pedersen NP, Sabsevitz DS, Block C, Dickey AS, Alwaki A, Kheder A. Cognitive and emotional mapping with SEEG. Frontiers in Neurology. 2021;**12**:627981. DOI: 10.3389/fneur.2021.627981

[57] Ritaccio AL, Brunner P, Schalk G. Electrical stimulation mapping of the brain: Basic principles and emerging alternatives. Journal of Clinical Neurophysiology. 2018;**35**(2):86–97. DOI: 10.1097/WNP.0000000000000440

[58] Rachidi I, Minotti L, Martin G, Hoffmann D, Bastin J, David O, Kahane P. The Insula: A Stimulating Island of

the Brain. Brain Sciences. 2021;**11**(11):1533. DOI: 10.3390/brainsci11111533

[59] Munakomi S, Das JM Epilepsy surgery. [Updated 2023 Aug 14]. In: StatPearls [Internet]. Treasure Island (FL): StatPearls Publishing; 2025-. Available from: https://www.ncbi.nlm.nih.gov/books/NBK562151/ [Accessed: 2025-November-13]

[60] Consales A, Cognolato E, Pacetti M, Mancardi MM, Tortora D, Di Perna G, Piatelli G, Nobili L. Magnetic resonance-guided laser interstitial thermal therapy (MR-gLiTT) in pediatric epilepsy surgery: State of the art and presentation of giannina gaslini children's hospital (Genoa, Italy) series. Frontiers in Neurology. 2021;**12**:739034. DOI: 10.3389/fneur.2021.739034

[61] Rieke V, Butts Pauly K. MR thermometry. Journal of Magnetic Resonance Imaging. 2008;**27**(2):376–390. DOI: 10.1002/jmri.21265

[62] Truong VT, Tayah T, Bouthillier A, Nguyen DK. Anterior corpus callosotomy in multistep invasive monitoring and surgery for atonic seizures. Epilepsy & Behavior Case Reports. 2014;**2**:11–14. DOI: 10.1016/j.ebcr.2013.12.003

[63] Sheikh K, Miller D, Blake R, Smith L, Conrad S, Sokol D, et al. Using magnetic resonance-guided laser interstitial thermal therapy corpus callosotomy to lateralize a seizure focus for staged surgical approach. Exploration of Neuroscience. 2024;**3**:198–206

[64] DiLorenzo DJ, Falowski SM, Wallace DJ, Corley JA, Fogg LF, Smith MC, Rossi MA, Balabanov AJ, Byrne RW. Intracranial monitoring and resective epilepsy surgery: Preoperative predictors of nonprogression to therapeutic surgery and long-term outcomes. International Journal of Academic Medicine. 2017;**3**(1):31–43. DOI: 10.4103/2455-5568.209856

[65] Warsi NM, Mohammad AH, Zhang F, Wong SM, Yan H, Mansouri A, Ibrahim GM. Electrocorticography-guided resection enhances postoperative seizure freedom in low-grade tumor-associated epilepsy: A Systematic Review and Meta-Analysis. Neurosurgery. 2023;**92**(1):18–26. DOI: 10.1227/neu.0000000000002182

[66] Yao P-S, Zheng S-F, Wang F, Kang D-Z, Lin Y-X. Surgery guided with intraoperative electrocorticography in patients with low-grade glioma and refractory seizures. Journal of Neurosurgery. 2018;**128**(3):840–845. DOI: 10.3171/2016.11.JNS161296

[67] Ravat S, Iyer V, Panchal K, Muzumdar D, Kulkarni A. Surgical outcomes in patients with intraoperative Electrocorticography (EcoG) guided epilepsy surgery-experiences of a tertiary care centre in India. International Journal of Surgery. 2016;**36**(Pt B):420–428. DOI: 10.1016/j.ijsu.2016.02.047

[68] Johnson H, Vestal ML, Husain AM. A novel technique for intraoperative mapping of the Somatosensory Cortex. World Neurosurgery. 2024;**188**:170–176. DOI: 10.1016/j.wneu.2024.05.118

[69] Cedzich C, Taniguchi M, Schäfer S, Schramm J. Somatosensory evoked potential phase reversal and direct motor cortex stimulation during surgery in and around the central region. Neurosurgery. 1996;**38**(5):962–970.

DOI: 10.1097/00006123-199605000-00023

[70] Ortiz KJ, Hawayek MI, Middlebrooks EH, Sabsevitz DS, Garcia DP, Quinones-Hinojosa A, Chaichana KL. Intraoperative direct stimulation identification and preservation of critical white matter tracts during brain surgery. World Neurosurgery. 2021;**146**:64–74. DOI: 10.1016/j.wneu.2020.10.100

[71] Roca E, Pallud J, Guerrini F, Panciani PP, Fontanella M, Spena G. Stimulation-related intraoperative seizures during awake surgery: A review of available evidences. Neurosurgical Review. 2020;**43**(1):87–93. DOI: 10.1007/s10143-019-01214-0

[72] Uribe A, Zuleta-Alarcon A, Kassem M, Sandhu GS, Bergese SD. Intraoperative seizures: Anesthetic and antiepileptic drugs. Current Pharmaceutical Design. 2018;**23**(42):6524–6532. DOI: 10.2174/1381612823666171024154026

[73] Miziak B, Borowicz-Reutt K, Rola R, Blaszczyk B, Czuczwar M, Czuczwar SJ. The prophylactic use of antiepileptic drugs in patients scheduled for neurosurgery. Current Pharmaceutical Design. 2018;**23**(42):6411–6427. DOI: 10.2174/1381612823666171027125408

[74] Alvi MA, Kwon BK, Hejrati N, et al. Accuracy of intraoperative neuromonitoring in the diagnosis of intraoperative neurological decline in the setting of spinal surgery—A systematic review and meta-analysis. Global Spine Journal. 2024;**14**(3_suppl):105S–149S. DOI: 10.1177/21925682231196514

[75] Chang SH, Park YG, Kim DH, Yoon SY. Monitoring of motor and somatosensory evoked potentials during spine surgery: Intraoperative changes and postoperative outcomes. Annals of Rehabilitation Medicine. 2016;**40**(3):470–480. DOI: 10.5535/arm.2016.40.3.470

[76] Stone SS, Rutka JT. Utility of neuronavigation and neuromonitoring in epilepsy surgery. Neurosurgical Focus. 2008;**25**(3):E17. DOI: 10.3171/FOC/2008/25/9/E17

[77] MacDonald DB, Simon MV, Nuwer MR. Neurophysiology during epilepsy surgery. Handbook of Clinical Neurology. 2022;**186**:103–121. DOI: 10.1016/B978-0-12-819826-1.00017-X

[78] Young CC, Williams JR, Feroze AH, McGrath M, Ravanpay AC, Ellenbogen RG, Ojemann JG, Hauptman JS. Pediatric functional hemispherectomy: Operative techniques and complication avoidance. Neurosurgical Focus. 2020;**48**(4):E9. DOI: 10.3171/2020.1.FOCUS19889

[79] McGovern RA, N V Moosa A, Jehi L, Busch R, Ferguson L, Gupta A, Gonzalez-martinez J, Wyllie E, Najm I, Bingaman WE. Hemispherectomy in adults and adolescents: Seizure and functional outcomes in 47 patients. Epilepsia. 2019;**60**(12):2416–2427. DOI: 10.1111/epi.16378

[80] Hertz-Pannier L, Chiron C, Jambaqué I, Renaux-kieffer V, de Moortele Pf V, Delalande O, Fohlen M, Brunelle F, Le Bihan D. Late plasticity for language in a child's non-dominant hemisphere: A pre- and post-surgery fMRI study. Brain. 2002;**125**(2): 361–372. DOI: 10.1093/brain/awf020

[81] Asadi-Pooya AA, Nei M, Sharan A, Sperling MR. Historical risk factors associated with seizure outcome after

surgery for drug-resistant mesial temporal lobe epilepsy. World Neurosurgery. 2016;**89**:78–83. DOI: 10.1016/j.wneu.2016.02.023

[82] Lee S-A, Yim SB, Lim YM, Kang JK, Lee JK. Factors predicting seizure outcome of anterior temporal lobectomy for patients with mesial temporal sclerosis. Seizure. 2006;**15** (6):397–404. DOI: 10.1016/j.seizure.2006.05.003

[83] Kerezoudis P, Parisi V, Marsh WR, Kaufman TJ, Lehman VT, Worrell GA, Miller KJ, Van Gompel JJ. Surgical outcomes of laser interstitial thermal therapy for temporal lobe epilepsy: Systematic review and meta-analysis. World Neurosurgery. 2020;**143**: 527–536.e3. DOI: 10.1016/j.wneu.2020.07.194

[84] Rugg-Gunn F, Miserocchi A, McEvoy A. Epilepsy surgery. Practical Neurology. 2020;**20**(1):4–14. DOI: 10.1136/practneurol-2019-002192

[85] Noe K, Sulc V, Wong-Kisiel L, Wirrell E, Van Gompel JJ, Wetjen N, Britton J, So E, Cascino GD, Marsh WR, Meyer F, Horinek D, Giannini C, Watson R, Brinkmann BH, Stead M, Worrell GA. Long-term outcomes after nonlesional extratemporal lobe epilepsy surgery. JAMA Neurology. 2013;**70** (8):1003–1008. DOI: 10.1001/jamaneurol.2013.209

[86] Sanders MW, Van der Wolf I, Jansen FE, Aronica E, Helmstaedter C, Racz A, Surges R, Grote A, Becker AJ, Rheims S, Catenoix H, Duncan JS, De Tisi J, Jacques TS, Cross JH, Kalviainen R, Rauramaa T, Chassoux F, Devaux BC, Di Gennaro G, Esposito V, Bodi I, Honavar M, Bien CG, Cloppenborg T, Coras R, Hamer HM, Marusic P, Kalina A, Pieper T, Kudernatsch M, Hartlieb TS, Von Oertzen TJ, Aichholzer M, Dorfmuller G, Chipaux M, Noachtar S, Kaufmann E, Schulze-Bonhage A, Scheiwe CF, Özkara C, Grunwald T, Koenig K, Guerrini R, Barba C, Buccoliero AM, Giordano F, Rosenow F, Menzler K, Garbelli R, Deleo F, Krsek P, Straka B, Arzimanoglou AA, Toulouse J, Van Paesschen W, Theys T, Pimentel J, De Amorim IM L, Specchio N, De Palma L, Feucht M, Scholl T, Roessler K, Toledano Delgado R, Gil-Nagel A, Raicevic S, Ristic AJ, Schijns O, Beckervordersandforth J, San Antonio-Arce V, Rumia J, Blumcke I, Braun KP. As the European Epilepsy Brain Bank Consortium (EEBB). Outcome of epilepsy surgery in MRI-Negative patients without histopathologic abnormalities in the resected tissue. Neurology. 2024;**102**(4):e208007 DOI: 10.1212/WNL.0000000000208007

[87] Donos C, Breier J, Friedman E, Rollo P, Johnson J, Moss L, Thompson S, Thomas M, Hope O, Slater J, Tandon N. Laser ablation for mesial temporal lobe epilepsy: Surgical and cognitive outcomes with and without mesial temporal sclerosis. Epilepsia. 2018;**59** (7):1421–1432. Epub 2018 Jun 12. Erratum in: Epilepsia. 2018 Nov;59 (11):2166. DOI: 10.1111/epi.14585. DOI: 10.1111/epi.14443

[88] Mehvari Habibabadi J, Moein H, Basiratnia R, Badihian S, Zaki B, Manouchehri N, Zare M, Barekatain M, Rahimian E, Mehvari Habibabadi A, Moein P, Aghakhani Y, Amina S, Lhatoo S. Outcome of lesional epilepsy surgery: Report of the first comprehensive epilepsy program in Iran. Neurology Clinical Practice. 2019;**9**(4):286–295. DOI: 10.1212/CPJ.0000000000000627

[89] Všianský V, Brázdil M, Rektor I, Doležalová I, Kočvarová J, Strýček O, Hemza J, Chrastina J, Brichtová E,

Horák O, Mužlayová P, Hermanová M, Hendrych M, Pail M. Twenty-five years of epilepsy surgery at a Central European comprehensive epilepsy center—Trends in intervention delay and outcomes. Epilepsia Open. 2023;**8**(3):991–1001. DOI: 10.1002/epi4.12769

[90] Ahmed S, Nadeem ZA, Kamran U, Ashfaq H, Ashraf H, Ashraf M, Agarwal A, Farooq M. Magnetic Resonance-Guided Laser Interstitial Thermal Therapy in the Management of Hypothalamic Hamartomas: A Systematic Review and Meta-Analysis. World Neurosurgery. 2024;**190**:463–469.e6. DOI: 10.1016/j.wneu.2024.08.009

[91] Barot N, Batra K, Zhang J, Klem ML, Castellano J, Gonzalez-Martinez J, Bagic A. Surgical outcomes between temporal, extratemporal epilepsies and hypothalamic hamartoma: Systematic review and meta-analysis of MRI-guided laser interstitial thermal therapy for drug-resistant epilepsy. Journal of Neurology, Neurosurgery & Psychiatry. 2022;**93**(2):133–143. DOI: 10.1136/jnnp-2021-326185

[92] Hagemann A, Bien CG, Kalbhenn T, Hopf JL, Grewe P. Epilepsy surgery in extratemporal vs temporal lobe epilepsy: changes in surgical volumes and seizure outcome between 1990 and 2017. Neurology. 2022;**98**(19):e1902–e1912. DOI: 10.1212/WNL.0000000000200194

[93] Fisher R, Salanova V, Witt T, Worth R, Henry T, Gross R, Oommen K, Osorio I, Nazzaro J, Labar D, Kaplitt M, Sperling M, Sandok E, Neal J, Handforth A, Stern J, DeSalles A, Chung S, Shetter A, Bergen D, Bakay R, Henderson J, French J, Baltuch G, Rosenfeld W, Youkilis A, Marks W, Garcia P, Barbaro N, Fountain N, Bazil C, Goodman R, McKhann G, Babu Krishnamurthy K, Papavassiliou S, Epstein C, Pollard J, Tonder L, Grebin J, Coffey R, Graves N; SANTE Study Group. Electrical stimulation of the anterior nucleus of thalamus for treatment of refractory epilepsy. Epilepsia. 2010;**51**(5):899–908. DOI: 10.1111/j.1528-1167.2010.02536.x

[94] Salanova V, Sperling MR, Gross RE, Irwin CP, Vollhaber JA, Giftakis JE, Fisher RS. The SANTÉ study at 10 years of follow-up: Effectiveness, safety, and sudden unexpected death in epilepsy. Epilepsia. 2021;**62**(6):1306–1317. DOI: 10.1111/epi.16895

[95] Ryvlin P, So EL, Gordon CM, Hesdorffer DC, Sperling MR, Devinsky O, Bunker MT, Olin B, Friedman D. Long-term surveillance of SUDEP in drug-resistant epilepsy patients treated with VNS therapy. Epilepsia. 2018;**59**(3):562–572. DOI: 10.1111/epi.14002

[96] Kossoff EH, Al-macki N, Cervenka MC, Kim HD, Liao J, Megaw K, Nathan JK, Raimann X, Rivera R, Wiemer-kruel A, Williams E, Zupec-kania BA. What are the minimum requirements for ketogenic diet services in resource-limited regions? Recommendations from the International League Against Epilepsy Task Force for Dietary Therapy. Epilepsia. 2015;**56**(9):1337–1342. DOI: 10.1111/epi.13039

[97] van der Louw E, van den Hurk D, Neal E, Leiendecker B, Fitzsimmon G, Dority L, Thompson L, Marchió M, Dudzińska M, Dressler A, Klepper J, Auvin S, Cross JH. Ketogenic diet guidelines for infants with refractory epilepsy. European Journal of Paediatric Neurology. 2016;**20**(6):798–809. DOI: 10.1016/j.ejpn.2016.07.009

[98] Kossoff EH, Zupec-kania BA, Auvin S, Ballaban-gil KR, Christina

Bergqvist AG, Blackford R, Buchhalter JR, Caraballo RH, Cross JH, Dahlin MG, Donner EJ, Guzel O, Jehle RS, Klepper J, Kang H-C, Lambrechts DA, Liu YMC, Nathan JK, Nordli Jr DR, Pfeifer HH, Rho JM, Scheffer IE, Sharma S, Stafstrom CE, Thiele EA, Turner Z, Vaccarezza MM, van der Louw EJTM, Veggiotti P, Wheless JW, Wirrell EC. Practice Committee of the Child Neurology Society. Optimal clinical management of children receiving dietary therapies for epilepsy: Updated recommendations of the International Ketogenic Diet Study Group. Epilepsia Open. 2018;**3**(2):175–192. DOI: 10.1002/epi4.12225

[99] van der Louw E, Aldaz V, Harvey J, Roan M, van den Hurk D, Cross JH, Auvin S. Optimal clinical management of children receiving ketogenic parenteral nutrition: A clinical practice guide. Developmental Medicine & Child Neurology. 2020;**62**(1):48–56. DOI: 10.1111/dmcn.14306

[100] Cervenka MC, Wood S, Bagary M, Balabanov A, Bercovici E, Brown M-G, Devinsky O, Di Lorenzo C, Doherty CP, Felton E, Healy LA, Klein P, Kverneland M, Lambrechts D, Langer J, Nathan J, Munn J, Nguyen P, Phillips M, Roehl K, Tanner A, Williams C, Zupec-Kania B. International recommendations for the management of adults treated with ketogenic diet therapies. Neurology Clinical Practice. 2021;**11**(5):385–397. DOI: 10.1212/CPJ.0000000000001007

[101] Martin-mcgill KJ, Bresnahan R, Levy RG, Cooper PN. Ketogenic diets for drug-resistant epilepsy. The Cochrane Database of Systematic Reviews. 2020;**6**(6):CD001903. DOI: 10.1002/14651858.CD001903.pub5

[102] Zuper-Kania B, Vanatta L, Johnson M. Ketogenic Diet Therapies for Neurological Disorders Pocket Guide. 5th ed. Santa Monica, CA: Charlie Foundation; 2019. Available from: https://www.bethzupeckania.com/product-page/pocket-guide-ketogenic-diet-therapies-for-neurological-disorders

[103] KetoDietCalculator Z-KB: Calculating Ketogenic Meals. Updated 5-30-21. Available from: https://charliefoundation.org/how-to-calculate-ketogenic-diets/ [Accessed: 2025-June-10]

[104] Pack AM. The association between antiepileptic drugs and bone disease. Epilepsy Currents. 2003;**3**(3):91–95. DOI: 10.1046/j.1535-7597.2003.03306.x

Section 4

Updates in Allergic Rhinitis

Chapter 5

Allergic Rhinitis

Kubra Yırgın and Mehmet Halil Celiksoy

Abstract

Rhinitis is an inflammation of the nasal mucosa. Allergic rhinitis, on the contrary, is an inflammation of the nose caused by an IgE-mediated reaction. Allergic rhinitis affects 2% to 25% of children, while the prevalence in adults ranges from 1% to 40%. Classic symptoms of allergic rhinitis include sneezing, nasal itching, runny nose, and nasal congestion. These symptoms are often accompanied by eye-related issues such as redness and itching. Allergic rhinitis can impact children's sleep quality, quality of life, and academic performance. Asthma is also present in 15% to 38% of patients with allergic rhinitis. In addition, moderate to severe allergic rhinitis can complicate asthma control.

Keywords: allergic rhinitis, allergy, atopy, children, rhinitis, childhood

1. Introduction

Allergic rhinitis (AR) is one of the most common chronic disorders, characterized by IgE-mediated inflammation of the nasal mucosa. The disease manifests with symptoms such as sneezing, nasal itching, rhinorrhea, and nasal obstruction. While AR significantly impairs quality of life, it also leads to school absenteeism and loss of work productivity. In moderate-to-severe forms, persistent symptoms despite treatment can disrupt sleep quality and cause additional problems such as impaired concentration, learning difficulties, and depression [1]. Therefore, AR should not be regarded merely as a "nasal disease" but rather as a systemic condition that impacts general health status and societal productivity. Given the nonspecific nature of symptoms, it is important to note that AR may often be misdiagnosed or undertreated, potentially leading to chronicity. As AR can also serve as a precursor to lower airway diseases such as asthma, early diagnosis and appropriate management are of particular importance [2]. The pathogenesis of AR involves the interplay of genetic predisposition, exposure to environmental allergens, epithelial barrier dysfunction, and a T helper 2 (Th2)-driven immune response. Its prevalence has been increasing, particularly in industrialized countries, in recent decades [1, 3].

The prevalence of AR in childhood varies across countries but is generally reported to be between 10% and 40% [4, 5]. Factors contributing to this high prevalence include air pollution, climate change, and lifestyle modifications. AR frequently coexists with comorbidities such as asthma, conjunctivitis, and sinusitis, thus affecting not only the upper airways but the entire respiratory tract, and is therefore considered a systemic disease [6]. In recent years, therapeutic strategies have extended beyond symptomatic management, with allergen immunotherapy and biologic agents emerging as disease-modifying approaches. Moreover, advances in molecular allergy diagnostics and individualized, patient-centered treatment protocols have gained increasing importance [7, 8].

2. Definition and terminology

AR is an inflammatory disease of the nasal mucosa that develops as a result of an immunoglobulin E (IgE)-mediated type I hypersensitivity reaction. Typical symptoms include rhinorrhea, nasal congestion, sneezing episodes, and nasal itching, often accompanied by ocular symptoms such as itching and tearing. These manifestations usually occur within minutes after allergen exposure and may resolve within hours or persist as a late-phase reaction. [1]

Two key elements define AR:

- Allergen exposure
- Inflammation mediated by specific IgE

For diagnosis, in addition to clinical symptoms, it is important to demonstrate allergen sensitization using objective tests, such as skin prick testing or the measurement of specific IgE levels [9, 10].

2.1 Terminology

- **Allergic rhinitis (AR):** A form of rhinitis triggered by an IgE-mediated mechanism.
- **Seasonal allergic rhinitis (SAR):** A condition triggered by aeroallergens such as pollen during spring and summer, commonly associated with sensitivity to grasses, trees, and weeds.
- **Perennial allergic rhinitis (PAR):** A condition characterized by year-round symptoms, typically caused by indoor allergens such as house dust mites, mold, and animal dander [10].

According to the AR and its impact on asthma (ARIA) guidelines, AR is classified by symptom frequency and duration:

- **Intermittent AR:** Symptoms are present for less than four days per week or for fewer than four consecutive weeks.
- **Persistent AR:** Symptoms are present for ≥4 days per week and for ≥4 weeks.

In addition, disease severity is graded as “mild” or “moderate-to-severe” [5].

3. Epidemiology and risk factors

3.1 Epidemiology

AR is among the most prevalent chronic conditions worldwide, with particularly high prevalence in children and young adults. According to the International Study of Asthma and Allergies in Childhood (ISAAC), the prevalence of allergic rhinoconjunctivitis was reported as 8.5% in children aged 6–7 years and 14.6% in those aged 13–14 years [11]. Large-scale meta-analyses have reported a lifetime prevalence of AR in children of approximately 19.9% [12]. In industrialized countries, prevalence ranges between 30% and 40% in children [13]. While rates are higher in Canada, the United States, and European countries, reported prevalence remains lower in developing countries, although it is increasing. This disparity is largely attributed to differences in diagnostic resources, environmental exposures, and genetic backgrounds. Over the past two decades, a global upward trend in AR prevalence has been observed, largely driven by environmental factors such as air pollution, climate change, lifestyle modifications, and reduced microbial exposure [14–17].

3.2 Risk factors

The interaction of genetic predisposition and environmental factors plays a key role in the development of AR.

Genetic predisposition: A family history of atopy is strongly associated with AR. Genes involved in IgE regulation, particularly those located within the MHC region on chromosome 6, have been implicated [18–20].

Environmental allergen exposure: Early and intense exposure to aeroallergens such as pollen, house dust mites, animal dander, mold, and cockroach allergens facilitates sensitization [21].

Air pollution: Diesel exhaust particles, ozone, and nitrogen dioxide impair epithelial barrier integrity, facilitating allergen penetration. Airborne particulate matter (PM2.5, PM10) is known to exacerbate AR symptoms [15, 18, 21].

Climate change: Rising temperatures and elevated carbon dioxide levels enhance pollen production and allergenic protein content. Extended pollen seasons and increased pollen loads intensify the duration and severity of symptoms [15,16].

Urbanization: Indoor air pollution, tobacco smoke, chemical exposure, and inadequate ventilation contribute to AR risk in childhood. Conversely, children raised in rural environments have a lower prevalence of AR, a phenomenon explained by greater microbial diversity and the hygiene hypothesis [14, 15].

Diet and microbiota: Within the framework of the hygiene hypothesis, insufficient microbial stimulation in early life increases susceptibility to atopic diseases. A Western diet, characterized by low fiber and high sugar intake, is associated with dysbiosis and heightened inflammation. Early antibiotic use, cesarean delivery, and reduced microbial exposures further elevate the risk [14, 19].

Other factors:

- Passive exposure to cigarette smoke

- Coexisting atopic disorders, such as asthma and atopic dermatitis
- Male sex (in childhood), obesity, and cesarean delivery [19–21].

4. Pathogenesis

AR is characterized by an IgE-mediated type I hypersensitivity response of the immune system to aeroallergens. Its pathogenesis involves a complex sequence of immune processes that include both early- and late-phase reactions.

4.1 Immunological processes

4.1.1 Sensitization phase:

AR arises from an abnormal immune response to allergens. Antigens that are normally tolerated in healthy individuals provoke hypersensitivity in atopic subjects. During the initial allergen exposure, antigen-presenting cells (dendritic cells) capture the allergen and migrate to regional lymph nodes in the nasal mucosa. Here, the allergen is presented to naïve CD4+ T cells, which subsequently differentiate into Th2 cells. These Th2 cells secrete cytokines such as IL-4, IL-5, and IL-13, which stimulate B cells to produce allergen-specific IgE. The IgE antibodies bind to Fc ε RI receptors on mast cells [22].

4.1.2 Early-phase reaction:

Upon re-exposure to the allergen, IgE-coated mast cells are activated, releasing both preformed and newly synthesized mediators, including histamine, tryptase, prostaglandin D2 (PGD2), and leukotrienes C4/D4/E4. These mediators induce vasodilation, increased mucus secretion, enhanced vascular permeability, sensory nerve stimulation (itching, sneezing), and bronchoconstriction, giving rise to the characteristic symptoms [21].

4.1.3 Late-phase reaction:

This phase develops four to eight hours after allergen exposure and involves the recruitment of eosinophils, basophils, T cells, and monocytes to the site of inflammation. Cytokines and chemokines such as IL-5, IL-9, and eotaxin enhance eosinophil recruitment. Eosinophil degranulation causes mucosal damage and initiates tissue remodeling [22, 23]. Clinically, nasal congestion, hyperreactivity, and increased sensitivity to stimuli predominate in this phase.

4.2 Epithelial barrier dysfunction

The nasal epithelium normally provides a physical barrier. However, allergens and environmental factors such as air pollution can disrupt epithelial tight junction proteins (e.g. occludin, claudin). This disruption facilitates allergen penetration and immune activation [24, 25]. Moreover, epithelial cells release "alarmins" such as TSLP, IL-25, and IL-33, which promote Th2 differentiation and activate type 2 innate lymphoid cells (ILC2), thereby amplifying the allergic response [22, 24, 26, 27].

4.3 Molecular and genetic factors

Filaggrin mutations contribute to impaired epithelial integrity [28]. Genetic variants, such as HLA-DQ and HLA-DRB1, influence antigen presentation and IgE production. In addition, Toll-like receptor (TLR) polymorphisms may affect allergen recognition and innate immune responses [21].

4.4 Microbiota and type 2 inflammation

Reduced microbial diversity in the nasal mucosa may impair immune tolerance. Particularly in childhood, antibiotic exposure and growth in overly sterile environments can diminish microbial variety. The immunopathogenesis of AR is dominated by a Th2-skewed immune response, with IL-4, IL-5, and IL-13 driving eosinophilic inflammation [29, 30].

5. Phenotypes and endotypes of rhinitis

Although AR is diagnosed based on symptoms and evidence of allergic sensitization, the clinical course and treatment response display significant heterogeneity. Therefore, the disease should be classified not only diagnostically but also by phenotypes and endotypes. A phenotype refers to the observable clinical characteristics of the disease (duration, severity, age, comorbidities). An endotype describes the underlying immunological and molecular mechanisms and is crucial for defining therapeutic targets. This distinction has become particularly important with the advent of immunomodulatory treatments such as allergen immunotherapy and biologic agents [31].

5.1 Major clinical phenotypes of AR

5.1.1 Classification by duration (ARIA criteria)

The ARIA classification, supported by the World Health Organization, is the most widely adopted system, categorizing AR by symptom duration and severity:

- **Intermittent AR:** Symptoms are present for fewer than 4 days per week or fewer than 4 weeks per year.

- **Persistent AR:** Symptoms are present for ≥4 days per week and for ≥4 consecutive weeks [21, 32].

5.1.2 Classification by severity

Mild AR is defined by the absence of sleep disturbances, impairment of daily activities, school or work performance, and social functioning. In contrast, moderate-to-severe AR is characterized by the presence of at least one of the following: sleep disturbances, impaired daytime performance, social restrictions, or bothersome symptoms [21, 32]. AR classification according to symptom duration and severity is shown in **Figure 1** [5].

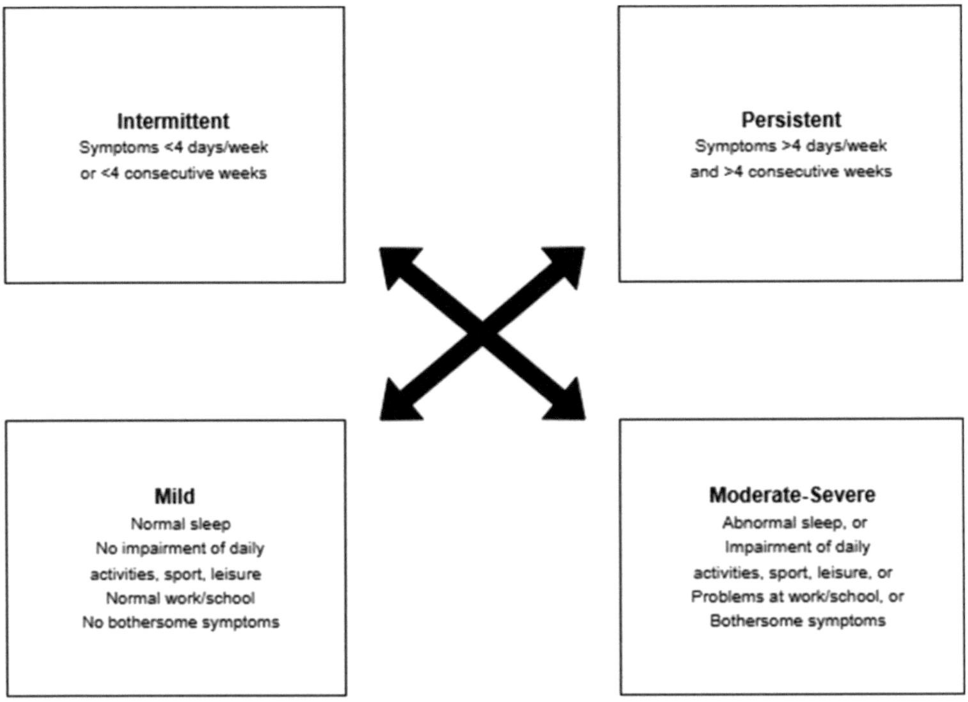

Figure 1.
Classification of AR according to symptom duration and severity[5].

5.1.3 Polysensitized versus monosensitized cases

Polysensitized patients exhibit sensitization to multiple allergens. Symptoms may persist year-round or fluctuate seasonally. Diagnosis and management can be complex, particularly in allergen selection for immunotherapy. Monosensitized patients are sensitized to a single allergen, often seen in SAR. Treatment response is generally more predictable, and immunotherapy is easier to plan.

5.1.4 Symptom-based phenotyping

AR can be classified based on predominant symptom profiles. The most common symptoms are rhinorrhea, nasal obstruction, sneezing, and itching. However, symptom intensity varies: the rhinorrhea/sneezing-dominant phenotype is often linked to histamine release and typically associated with pollen allergy. The congestion-dominant phenotype is more closely associated with perennial allergens such as house dust mites and molds. Here, both early and late-phase inflammatory responses are involved; histamine drives edema and rhinorrhea, while leukotrienes, prostaglandins, TNF-α, and IL-4 contribute to nasal obstruction [33, 34].

Symptom-based phenotyping is important for personalizing treatment strategies: antihistamines are more effective in rhinorrhea/sneezing-dominant phenotypes, whereas intranasal corticosteroids (INCS) are preferred in congestion-dominant phenotypes. Symptom persistence (intermittent vs. persistent) further guides treatment intensity and duration [21].

5.1.5 Local AR

Local AR (LAR) is a phenotype characterized by local nasal IgE production despite negative systemic IgE. These patients present with typical AR symptoms, negative skin prick and serum-specific IgE tests, but positive nasal provocation tests. LAR is an under-recognized subtype of AR, and management approaches largely overlap with those of classical AR [35, 36].

5.2 Immunological endotypes

5.2.1 Type 2 endotype (th2-driven)

The type 2 endotype encompasses mechanisms mediated by Th2 cells and can be divided into IgE-mediated and non-IgE-mediated pathways.

5.2.1.1 IgE-mediated type 2 endotype.

This is the most common form of rhinitis, characterized by IgE-mediated inflammation of the nasal mucosa in atopic individuals. Its pathogenesis involves allergen exposure, antigen presentation, and activation of Th2 responses, resulting in increased production of IL-4, IL-5, and IL-13, with subsequent IgE production, as well as mast cell and eosinophil activation [10].

5.2.1.2 Non-allergic eosinophilic rhinitis.

Non-Allergic Eosinophilic Rhinitis (NARES) is a non-IgE-mediated rhinitis subtype characterized by marked eosinophilic infiltration of the nasal mucosa despite negative systemic IgE. Elevated eosinophil counts in nasal secretions are a hallmark. Inflammatory mediators, such as eosinophil cationic protein (ECP) and major basic protein (MBP), are thought to drive symptoms and mucosal inflammation. NARES may be a precursor to asthma and nasal polyposis, thus warranting careful evaluation. Topical corticosteroids are generally effective in treatment [10, 37].

5.2.2 Non–type 2 endotype

This group is not dominated by the classical IgE-eosinophil axis. Inflammation may be neutrophilic, IgE levels are normal or negative, and skin prick tests are often negative. Triggers include vasomotor, gustatory, or hormonal factors [9]. These patients typically respond poorly to standard allergy treatments, and diagnosis and management are challenging due to nonspecific symptoms [38].

5.3 Clinical significance and therapeutic implications

The classification of AR into phenotypes and endotypes has direct implications for management. Type 2 phenotypes benefit from allergen immunotherapy and anti-IgE biologics. Non-type 2 patients may require intranasal anticholinergics or alternative therapies. INCS remain first-line for persistent, moderate-to-severe disease. In LAR cases, delayed diagnosis may postpone appropriate treatment. In conclusion, phenotype and endotype stratification form the basis of personalized diagnosis and treatment in AR. This classification is essential for predicting disease course, prognosis, and therapeutic response [21, 31, 39].

6. Clinical findings and comorbidities

6.1 Clinical symptoms

AR is characteristically manifested by typical symptoms that develop following exposure to allergens in the nasal mucosa. The clinical picture most frequently includes the following symptoms:

Major symptoms:

Sneezing attacks, usually more pronounced in the morning and after allergen exposure, are sequential and repetitive in nature. Nasal discharge (rhinorrhea) is watery and clear, commonly presenting as both anterior and postnasal drip. Nasal obstruction develops due to inflammation and mucosal edema, representing one of the most quality-of-life-limiting symptoms. Nasal itching often leads children to perform the upward rubbing motion of the nasal tip, known as the allergic salute.

Additional symptoms:

Ocular itching, redness, and tearing (typically bilateral and symmetric); itching in the throat and palate; dry cough due to postnasal drip; fatigue; attention deficit; impaired sleep quality; and a decreased sense of smell and taste may also occur [9, 21, 37, 40–44].

6.2 Physical examination findings

On physical examination, patients with AR often present with pale, edematous, or occasionally hyperemic nasal mucosa, accompanied by watery nasal discharge. Mouth breathing may be observed as a consequence of nasal obstruction. Characteristic findings also include dark periorbital circles ("allergic shiners"), conjunctival hyperemia, lower eyelid edema, and a transverse nasal crease caused by repetitive upward rubbing of the nose ("allergic salute"). In addition, turbinate hypertrophy is a feature in affected individuals [45, 46].

6.3 Age-specific clinical features

6.3.1 Infancy

AR is rare during infancy; however, eosinophilic mucositis may be observed in infants with an atopic history. More often, nonspecific nasal discharge and irritability may be present. It can be mistaken for gastroesophageal reflux [10, 47–49].

6.3.2 Preschool age

The most frequent symptom is nasal obstruction. Sleep problems, snoring, and attention difficulties are common [50]. The diagnosis of AR is often established at this age.

6.3.3 School-age children and adolescents

All typical symptoms (sneezing, rhinorrhea, itching) become clearly expressed. A decline in school performance, concentration difficulties, and social isolation may be observed [51]. Asthma and conjunctivitis frequently coexist.

6.3.4 Adults and the elderly

Symptoms may resemble classical AR, but age-related mucosal changes, olfactory loss, and drug side effects become more prominent. In older adults, symptoms may be milder, but concomitant diseases often complicate diagnosis [52].

6.4 Seasonal and periodic characteristics of symptoms

SAR occurs in relation to pollen seasons, with symptoms typically exacerbating during spring and summer [21]. PAR, on the contrary, is triggered by continuous exposure to indoor allergens such as house dust mites, animal dander, or mold [21]. Occupational AR develops as a result of exposure to specific allergens in the workplace, such as flour in bakery workers [53].

6.5 Impact of symptoms on patients

Sleep disruption due to nasal obstruction can result in daytime fatigue and sleep disturbances. Ocular symptoms, itching, and nasal discharge may limit social interactions. Particularly in younger age groups, learning difficulties and attention deficits can lead to reduced academic or occupational performance. Long-term symptoms have been linked to depression and anxiety [54, 55].

6.6 Comorbidities

AR is not merely a condition confined to the nasal mucosa; it is a disorder characterized by systemic inflammatory responses, potentially affecting multiple organ systems. Numerous allergic diseases, driven by a shared type-2 immune response, tend to coexist with AR.

Asthma:

Asthma is present in approximately 10%–40% of AR patients, while 60%–80% of individuals with asthma have concomitant AR [1, 5]. Treating AR improves asthma control and reduces the risk of exacerbations. The upper and lower airways share similar epithelial structures, with the same allergens triggering comparable cellular and cytokine responses. Nasal inflammation may enhance bronchial hyperreactivity.

Allergic conjunctivitis:

Characterized by itching, redness, and tearing, it is the most common comorbidity of AR, particularly intensified during pollen seasons in patients with SAR. INCS and antihistamines may improve both nasal and ocular symptoms [56, 57].

Sinusitis and nasal polyposis:
AR patients have an increased risk of chronic rhinosinusitis (CRS). Both polypoid (type-2 dominant) and non-polypoid CRS subtypes may coexist. Special attention should be given to aspirin-exacerbated respiratory disease (Samter's triad). Biologic agents (e.g. anti-IL-5, anti-IgE) have emerged as potential treatment options. [58, 59]

Sleep disorders:
Nasal obstruction, snoring, and mouth breathing significantly impair sleep quality. The risk of obstructive sleep apnea syndrome (OSAS) is increased. Daytime fatigue, attention problems, irritability, and reduced school or work performance are frequent. In children, hyperactivity and behavioral problems may develop [42, 50, 60].

Otitis media and eustachian tube dysfunction:
Otitis media (especially with effusion) is associated with nasopharyngeal edema and eustachian tube dysfunction. Adenoid hypertrophy exacerbates nasal obstruction and impairs sleep quality in children [58]. Appropriate AR treatment may reduce the incidence of these complications.

Atopic dermatitis and food allergies:
AR is more common in atopic individuals. In polysensitized patients, atopic dermatitis and food sensitivities may coexist with AR [61].

Gastroesophageal reflux:
Nasal obstruction can lead to mouth breathing and laryngeal irritation. AR and gastroesophageal reflux frequently coexist, though a causal relationship is not fully established [62]. Treating both conditions together significantly alleviates symptoms.

Allergic march and systemic atopy:
The allergic march describes the progression of atopic diseases that begin in early life and evolve into different clinical entities over time [63]:

- 0–2 years: Atopic dermatitis, food allergies [64].
- 2–5 years: Onset of AR [63].
- Over 5 years: Asthma, conjunctivitis, polyvalent atopic syndromes [65]

Early diagnosis and intervention may slow or even halt this progression [64].

7. Diagnostic approaches

The diagnosis of AR is established through a combination of typical symptoms, detailed medical history, physical examination, and tests demonstrating allergen sensitization. The aim of the diagnostic process is to demonstrate that the patient's symptoms result from an IgE-mediated response to a specific allergen.

7.1 Medical history

Medical history forms the cornerstone of diagnosis in AR. Particular attention should be paid to the type, severity, seasonality, and duration of symptoms, as well as potential exposure to common allergens such as animals, house dust, pollens, molds, or occupational agents. A family history of atopic diseases is an important contributing factor. The impact of symptoms on sleep quality and school or work performance should also be assessed. In addition, the presence of comorbid conditions, including asthma, conjunctivitis, or atopic dermatitis, as well as possible occupational exposures, must be carefully evaluated [37].

7.2 Physical examination

On physical examination, patients with AR frequently exhibit pale and edematous nasal mucosa accompanied by watery nasal discharge. Periorbital hyperpigmentation, also known as the allergic shiner, and a transverse crease on the nasal tip resulting from the repetitive allergic salute are characteristic findings. In addition, nasal endoscopy is a valuable tool for excluding structural abnormalities such as nasal polyps, septal deviation, foreign bodies, or tumors [66].

7.3 Allergy testing

1. **Skin prick test:**
   The skin prick test is the most widely used diagnostic method. It is performed with both negative and positive controls, and results are obtained within 15–20 minutes. Advantages include rapidity, cost-effectiveness, and high sensitivity. Antihistamine use may interfere with test results [67].

2. **Specific IgE testing (in vitro):**
   Serum allergen-specific IgE levels are measured. This method is preferred in patients for whom skin testing is not feasible (e.g. severe dermographism, extensive atopic dermatitis, or infants). ImmunoCAP is the most commonly used technique. Unlike the skin prick test, antihistamine use does not affect test results [67].

3. **Molecular allergy testing:**
   Assesses sensitization to specific allergen components. It enables differentiation between polysensitization and cross-reactivity and may guide decisions regarding immunotherapy [68].

7.4 Other diagnostic methods

Nasal cytology
Eosinophils can be demonstrated in nasal secretion samples, which is particularly useful in differentiating NARES. This method is reproducible, non-invasive, economical, and applicable for phenotyping [69, 70].

Nasal provocation test
This is indicated in cases of uncertain sensitization or when the clinical presentation and test results are incongruent. It is considered the gold standard for diagnosing LAR. The procedure involves the direct application of allergens to the nasal mucosa to provoke symptoms and is performed only in specialized centers [71].

Total IgE and eosinophil count
Not specific for AR diagnosis; however, elevated total IgE and eosinophilia are common in atopic individuals.

7.5 Advanced assessment and functional tests

7.5.1 Rhinomanometry and acoustic rhinometry

Provide objective measurements of nasal airflow and obstruction. These measurements are used to monitor mucosal changes before and after treatment [72].

7.5.2 Nasal endoscopy

Indicated for excluding structural abnormalities such as polyps, masses, or septal deviation; this approach is particularly valuable in treatment-resistant cases [73].

7.5.3 Olfactory testing

Used for the objective assessment of olfactory function, persistent AR may present with hyposmia or anosmia. Olfactory testing aids in treatment planning and disease monitoring, particularly in evaluating the impact of chronic inflammation on the olfactory epithelium [6, 74].

8. Differential diagnosis

AR may present with a clinical picture resembling many other nasal disorders characterized by similar symptoms. Ruling out these conditions during the diagnostic process is crucial to avoid misdiagnosis and inappropriate treatment [7].

8.1 Non-AR

Non-Allergic Rhinitis (NAR)

Develops through non-immunological mechanisms, generally not IgE-mediated. Although symptoms resemble AR, allergy test results are negative.

Subtypes include:

- Vasomotor rhinitis: Triggered by nonspecific stimuli such as odors, stress, alcohol, temperature changes, or cigarette smoke.
- Drug-induced rhinitis: Includes "rhinitis medicamentosa" caused by the overuse of decongestants; it is also associated with ACE inhibitors, oral contraceptives, aspirin, etc.
- Hormonal rhinitis: Observed during pregnancy or in cases of thyroid disorders.
- Atrophic rhinitis: Characterized by the thinning of the nasal mucosa and a foul-smelling discharge.

- Occupational rhinitis: Triggered by workplace exposures, sometimes IgE-mediated. [75]

NARES (non-AR with eosinophilia syndrome)
Allergy tests are negative, but nasal cytology demonstrates eosinophilia. Symptoms resemble AR, and nasal cytology is helpful in diagnosis [75].

8.2 Infectious rhinitis

Acute viral rhinitis (common cold)
Symptoms are short-lived (less than 10 days). Fever, sore throat, and systemic complaints are prominent. Nasal discharge is initially clear but may become mucopurulent.

Chronic rhinosinusitis
Characterized by nasal obstruction, mucopurulent discharge, facial pain, and olfactory dysfunction lasting more than 12 weeks. Diagnosis is established through nasal endoscopy and CT imaging [76].

8.3 Other differential diagnoses

Structural anomalies

- Nasal septal deviation
- Turbinate hypertrophy
- Nasal polyps (unilateral polyps should raise suspicion of a neoplasm).
- Adenoid hypertrophy [7]

Foreign bodies
Particularly in children, it causes unilateral foul-smelling discharge [77].

Nasopharyngeal tumors
Should be suspected in cases of unilateral nasal obstruction, bloody discharge, or atypical facial pain [7].

Cerebrospinal fluid (CSF) leak
Presents after trauma with unilateral watery discharge that worsens when leaning forward. Diagnosis can be confirmed by beta-2 transferrin assay [7].

Systemic diseases

- Granulomatosis with polyangiitis (Wegener's disease)
- Sarcoidosis
- Churg–Strauss syndrome (eosinophilic granulomatosis with polyangiitis)

These conditions are usually accompanied by systemic manifestations [7].

9. Treatment options

The primary goals of AR management are to control symptoms, modify the natural course of the disease, improve quality of life, and manage associated comorbidities. Treatment should be individualized, taking into account the duration and severity of symptoms, the presence of comorbid conditions, the allergen exposure profile, and patient preferences. Three main therapeutic approaches are emphasized in AR: allergen avoidance, pharmacotherapy, and allergen immunotherapy. Together, these strategies target both symptomatic control and immunological modulation of the disease.

9.1 Allergen avoidance and other non-pharmacological approaches

Allergen avoidance is particularly important for patients with symptoms attributable to a specific sensitization. Preventive measures against common aeroallergens, such as house dust mites, animal dander, pollens, molds, and cockroaches, may reduce disease severity. However, studies have demonstrated that these measures alone are insufficient for many patients and are more effective when combined with pharmacological therapy [78].

Nasal saline irrigation is also recommended as a non-pharmacological intervention. Saline rinses help physically remove allergen particles from the nasal mucosa, reduce mucus viscosity, and improve the efficacy of topical medications. While saline irrigation may provide sufficient relief in mild cases, it is most effective when used alongside pharmacotherapy in moderate to severe disease [79, 80].

9.2 Pharmacological treatment

Pharmacological treatment is used to quickly and effectively control the symptoms of AR. Treatment options vary depending on the severity and duration of the disease.

INCS represent the most effective therapeutic option in AR. By suppressing inflammation in the nasal mucosa, they act on both early- and late-phase allergic responses. Commonly used agents include fluticasone, mometasone, budesonide, and beclomethasone. INCS significantly reduce symptoms such as nasal obstruction, rhinorrhea, and sneezing. Adverse effects are usually mild, including local irritation, nasal dryness, and occasionally epistaxis. Systemic absorption is minimal, and even with long-term use, INCS maintain favorable safety profiles [81, 82].

Oral antihistamines, particularly second-generation non-sedating agents (e.g. desloratadine, fexofenadine, loratadine, levocetirizine), are suitable for patients with mild symptoms or those unwilling to use INCS. They control sneezing, rhinorrhea, and nasal itching via H1-receptor blockade. As their sedative effects are minimal, they can be used without impairing daily activities. However, their efficacy against nasal congestion is limited. [83]

Intranasal antihistamines (e.g. azelastine, olopatadine) provide rapid local symptom control and are particularly useful in mild-to-moderate disease or in patients unable to tolerate systemic antihistamines. Combination therapy with INCS may exert a synergistic effect [84, 85].

Leukotriene receptor antagonists (LTRAs), such as montelukast, are recommended, especially for patients with concomitant asthma. They reduce nasal obstruction and nocturnal symptoms by blocking leukotriene D4 receptors, thereby attenuating inflammation in both the upper and lower airways. However, their efficacy as monotherapy for AR is inferior to that of INCS. Rare psychiatric adverse effects associated with montelukast warrant cautious use [66, 84, 86].

Decongestants may provide short-term symptomatic relief. Topical agents, such as oxymetazoline, are effective when used for ≤3–5 days; however, prolonged use may cause rebound congestion (rhinitis medicamentosa). Systemic decongestants (e.g. pseudoephedrine) are restricted to selected patients due to potential adverse effects, including hypertension, tachycardia, and sleep disturbances [21, 66]. Systemic corticosteroids are reserved for severe, uncontrolled symptoms and should only be administered short term (3–5 days). Long-term use is discouraged due to risks such as osteoporosis, growth retardation, hypertension, and diabetes mellitus [87].

Cromolyn sodium, a mast cell stabilizer, is considered safe for sensitive populations such as children and pregnant women. Although its efficacy is limited, it may be valuable for prophylaxis [88]. Ipratropium bromide may be beneficial in cases where watery rhinorrhea is the predominant symptom. The doses of drugs used in AR according to age are provided in **Table 1** [21].

	Usual adult dose	**Usual pediatric dose**
	Oral antihistamines (second generation)	
Bilastine (Blexten)	1 tablet (20 mg) once daily	For children aged 4–11 years: 10 mg once daily (1 orodispersible tablet or 4 mL of oral solution). For children over 12 years of age: 1 tablet (20 mg) once daily.
Cetirizine (Reactine)	1–2 tablets (5 mg) once daily 1 tablet (10 mg) once daily	5–10 mL (1–2 teaspoons) once daily (children's formulation)
Desloratadine (Aerius)	1 tablet (5 mg) once daily	2.5–5 mL (0.5–1.0 teaspoons) once daily (children's formulation)
Fexofenadine (Allegra)	1 tablet (60 mg) every 12 hours (12-hour formulation). 1 tablet (120 mg), once daily (24-hour formulation).	Not currently indicated for children under 12 years of age
Loratadine (Claritin)	1 tablet (10 mg), once daily	5–10 mL (1–2 teaspoons) once daily (children's formulation)
Rupatadine (Rupall)	1 tablet (10 mg) once daily	For children aged 12 years and older: 1 tablet (10 mg) once daily. For children aged 2–11 years with a body weight of 10–25 kg, administer 2.5 mL (0.5 teaspoon) once daily. For children aged 2–11 years with a body weight greater than 25 kg: 5 mL (1.0 teaspoon) once daily.
	Intranasal corticosteroids	
Beclomethasone (Beconase)	1–2 sprays (50 μg/spray) EN, twice daily	1 spray (50 μg/spray) EN, twice daily

	Usual adult dose	Usual pediatric dose
Budesonide (Rhinocort)	2 sprays (64 µg/spray) EN once daily, or 1 spray EN twice daily	2 sprays (64 µg/spray) EN, once daily, or 1 spray EN, twice daily (do not exceed 256 µg)
Ciclesonide (Omnaris)	2 sprays (50 µg/spray) EN, once daily	Not indicated for children under 12 years of age
Fluticasone furoate (Avamys)	2 sprays (27.5 µg/spray) EN, once daily	1 spray (27.5 µg/spray) EN, once daily
Fluticasone propionate (Flonase)	2 sprays (50 µg/spray) of EN, once daily or every 12 hours (for severe rhinitis)	1–2 sprays (50 µg/spray) EN, once daily
Mometasone furoate (Nasonex)	2 sprays (50 µg/spray) EN, once daily	1 spray (50 µg/spray) EN, once daily
Triamcinolone acetonide (Nasacort)	2 sprays (55 µg/spray) EN, once daily	1 spray (55 µg/spray) EN, once daily
Combination intranasal corticosteroid/antihistamine nasal spray		
Fluticasone propionate/ azelastine hydrochloride (Dymista)	1 spray EN, twice daily	For children over 12 years of age: 1 spray in each nostril, twice daily. Not recommended for children under 12 years of age.
Olopatadine hydrochloride/ mometasone furoate monohydrate (Ryaltris)	2 sprays EN, twice daily	For children aged 6–11 years: 1 spray in each nostril, twice daily. For children over 12 years of age: 2 sprays in each nostril, twice daily.
Leukotriene receptor antagonists		
Montelukast	1 tablet (10 mg), once daily	Not currently approved for patients under 15 years of age

Table 1.
Overview of pharmacological treatment options for AR.

9.3 Treatment planning

The most widely used treatment algorithm for AR is provided by the ARIA guidelines. According to ARIA, treatment selection is guided by the frequency and severity of symptoms.

- For intermittent or mild symptoms, oral antihistamines or low-dose INCS are recommended.
- For persistent or moderate-to-severe disease, INCS are considered the first-line therapy.
- If necessary, intranasal antihistamines or LTRAs may be added to INCS.

Treatment response should be assessed within 2–4 weeks, with adjustments in dosage or therapeutic agents made accordingly [7]. In addition, a treatment algorithm for childhood AR was recently reported by the European Forum for Research and Education in Allergy and Airway Diseases (EUFOREA; see **Figure 2**) [47].

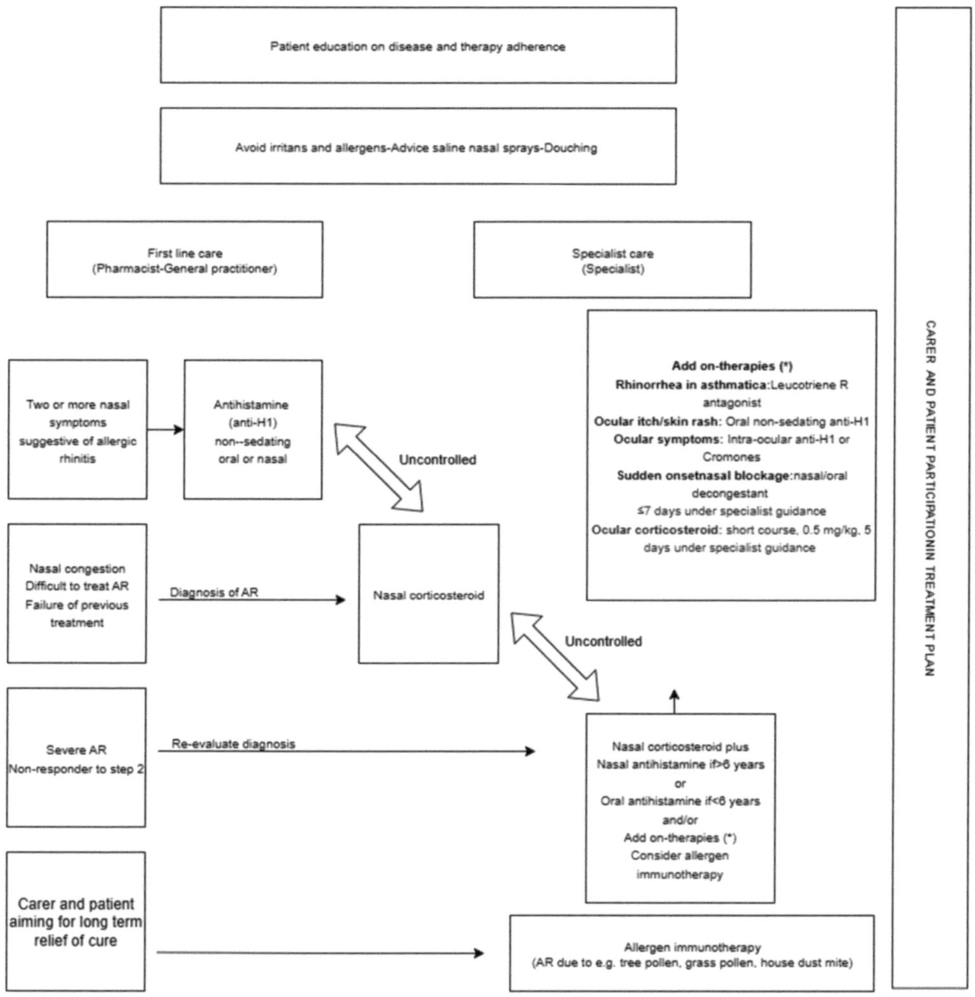

Figure 2.
Pediatric AR management algorithm.

10. Allergen avoidance strategies

Allergen avoidance constitutes a fundamental approach in the management of AR. In patients with confirmed sensitization to specific allergens, reducing exposure significantly contributes to symptom control [78]. However, allergen avoidance alone is usually insufficient; it is recommended to be used in combination with pharmacological therapy and/or immunotherapy.

10.1 House dust mites

House dust mites (*Dermatophagoides pteronyssinus* and *Dermatophagoides farinae*) are major triggers of PAR. They are particularly abundant in mattresses, pillows, carpets, duvets, and upholstered furniture. Recommended measures to reduce mite exposure include the following, though achieving a significant clinical impact is often difficult with single interventions [89–91]:

- Encasement of mattresses and pillows in mite-proof covers.
- Removal of dust-accumulating items, such as carpets, plush toys, and fabric curtains, from the bedroom.
- Weekly washing of bedding at 60°C.
- Maintaining indoor humidity below 50% (mites proliferate more actively under high humidity).
- Use of HEPA-filtered vacuum cleaners

Studies suggest that, when implemented in combination, these strategies can reduce overall indoor mite load and alleviate symptom severity.

10.2 Pollens

Pollen is the most common trigger of SAR. Preventive measures during the pollen season can be summarized as follows [92]:

- Avoiding outdoor exposure during periods of high pollen counts, especially during the morning hours (05:00–10:00).
- Showering and changing clothes after outdoor activities.
- Keeping windows closed and using air conditioning with filters at home and in cars.
- Use of pollen-filter masks, particularly for highly sensitive individuals.
- Monitoring pollen calendars and regional pollen concentration maps, and adjusting daily habits accordingly.

10.3 Mold spores

Molds (Alternaria, Cladosporium, etc.) are found both indoors and outdoors. Recommended preventive measures include [93]:

- Ensuring proper ventilation, especially in bathrooms.
- Eliminating sources of dampness (leaking pipes, humid walls).
- Using bleach-based cleaning products to remove mold.
- Avoiding indoor drying of laundry

However, in individuals sensitized to mold, there is insufficient evidence to confirm that these measures consistently improve symptom control [94].

10.4 Animals

Cat and dog dander are potent aeroallergen sources. For sensitized individuals, complete removal of the animal from the home is the ideal measure. However, since this is often not feasible, the following strategies are recommended [95, 96]:

- Restricting animal access to the bedroom.
- Use of HEPA-filter air purifiers
- Regular bathing and grooming of the animal.
- Reducing carpets and fabric-covered surfaces in the home.

Because animal allergens are small and adhere strongly to surfaces and air particles, exposure may persist for weeks, even after the animal has been removed from the household.

10.5 Cockroaches

Cockroach allergens are particularly prevalent in humid and crowded environments. Preventive strategies include eliminating food residues, ensuring regular cleaning and pest control, and sealing entry pathways such as cracks and ventilation openings [97, 98].

10.6 Tobacco smoke and other irritants

Tobacco smoke, passive smoking, and air pollution exacerbate AR symptoms [99, 100]. Avoidance of such irritants improves treatment outcomes. Passive exposure to tobacco smoke in children is associated with increased symptom severity, as well as a higher risk of comorbid asthma [100, 101]. For allergen avoidance strategies to be effective, they should be individualized, feasible, and sustainable. Moreover, these measures must be reinforced through patient education and, particularly in children, through active parental involvement.

11. Allergen-specific immunotherapy

Allergen-specific immunotherapy (AIT) is the only disease-modifying treatment modality targeting the pathogenesis of AR. AIT aims to induce immune tolerance through the controlled administration of gradually increasing doses of the causative allergen. Beyond alleviating symptoms, AIT may prevent the development of new sensitizations and the onset of comorbid asthma [102, 103].

11.1 Indications

AIT is indicated in patients with a confirmed diagnosis of AR and objectively demonstrated sensitization under the following conditions [103]:

- Presence of moderate-to-severe symptoms inadequately controlled with pharmacological therapy.

- Dependence on long-term pharmacological treatment and/or the occurrence of treatment-related adverse effects.

- Patient preference, particularly among those seeking a non-pharmacological, long-term solution.

- Desire to modify the natural course of the disease through immune tolerance induction.

For allergen immunotherapy (AIT) to be considered, there must be a clear clinical correlation between the patient's symptoms and the identified allergen sensitization.

11.2 Routes of administration

AIT can be administered through two primary methods:

1. Subcutaneous immunotherapy (SCIT)
This method involves allergen administration via subcutaneous injections. The protocol begins with weekly dose escalations (induction phase), followed by a maintenance phase with monthly injections. The total treatment duration is generally 3–5 years. SCIT is the most extensively studied method with the longest clinical experience, and its efficacy has been demonstrated against pollens, house dust mites, and cat dander.

2. Sublingual immunotherapy (SLIT)
This approach involves the administration of allergens in drop or tablet formulations under the tongue. SLIT can be self-administered at home, typically requiring daily intake. It has a more favorable safety profile, with fewer systemic adverse events [104]. SLIT is more widely used for pollen allergies due to the availability of licensed products. Given its convenience of at-home administration, patient adherence may be higher compared to SCIT.

11.3 Efficacy and safety

AIT is supported by numerous randomized controlled trials demonstrating its efficacy. Evidence indicates that AIT reduces symptom scores and medication use, prevents asthma development, and maintains its effectiveness for at least 2–3 years after the completion of therapy [102, 105, 106]. The most serious complication of SCIT is anaphylaxis, making physician supervision and access to emergency interventions mandatory during administration [107]. The most common adverse effects of SLIT include oral pruritus, throat irritation, and, less frequently, gastrointestinal symptoms [104, 107–109]. It is recommended that the first SLIT dose also be administered in a clinical setting.

11.4 Patient selection and contraindications

Patient selection for AIT requires careful consideration of several factors. A clearly defined IgE-mediated allergen sensitization with clinical correlation is essential, and the patient must be motivated and capable of adhering to the treatment protocol. Asthma should be well-controlled, as AIT is contraindicated in active or severe asthma. Caution is warranted in patients receiving beta-blockers or those with severe cardiovascular disease. Moreover, AIT is contraindicated in individuals with severe immunodeficiency, autoimmune disorders, or malignancy [103]. Importantly, AIT should not be initiated during pregnancy; however, if treatment was already initiated prior to conception and is well-tolerated, continuation may be considered.

12. Prognosis and follow-up

AR is generally a chronic and recurrent condition. If inadequately managed, symptoms can substantially impair quality of life, reduce school and work performance, and predispose patients to comorbidities such as sleep disorders, sinusitis, and asthma.

12.1 Natural course of the disease

The prognosis of AR varies between individuals. In most cases with childhood onset, symptoms persist into adulthood. While some individuals experience symptom reduction with age, complete remission is rare. In SAR, particularly pollen-induced cases, symptom duration often extends over time, and polysensitization may develop [110]. Patients with AR have a significantly increased risk of developing asthma compared to the healthy population. This association is explained by the concept of "united airway disease," as the upper and lower airways share similar immunological and anatomical characteristics. Consequently, inflammation originating in one part of the airway may eventually affect the other [111, 112]. For this reason, periodic monitoring with pulmonary function tests is recommended in pediatric patients to assess asthma development.

12.2 Evaluation of treatment response

The primary objective of AR management is symptom control and improvement in quality of life. Treatment response should be assessed through both subjective patient-reported outcomes and objective evaluations. Clinical improvement is typically expected within 2–4 weeks of initiating therapy [7]. In cases of insufficient response, treatment dosage, modality, and adherence should be reassessed, and comorbidities should be considered. In patients undergoing AIT, symptom improvement is usually observed within the first year; however, full therapeutic benefit may take 1–2 years to manifest [113, 114]. Long-term clinical benefits have also been demonstrated to persist after the completion of AIT.

12.3 Frequency and principles of follow-up

Follow-up schedules for patients with AR should be individualized according to disease severity, treatment response, and the presence of comorbidities. Annual evaluations may suffice for patients with mild, intermittent disease, whereas persistent or severe cases require more frequent follow-ups [7]. For refractory or atypical presentations, collaboration with allergy and otorhinolaryngology specialists is crucial. In pediatric patients, regular monitoring of growth and development, as well as early detection of comorbid conditions such as atopic dermatitis, food allergies, or asthma, is strongly recommended.

13. Management of treatment-resistant cases

In patients with treatment-resistant AR, it is essential to reassess the accuracy of the diagnosis, the adequacy of allergen avoidance strategies, treatment adherence, medication administration technique, and the presence of comorbidities (such as sinusitis, asthma, and gastroesophageal reflux). If necessary, advanced diagnostic tests and nasal endoscopy should be performed to evaluate for anatomical abnormalities.

13.1 Surgical interventions

For patients unresponsive to pharmacotherapy, surgical approaches (e.g. turbinate reduction, septoplasty, endoscopic sinus surgery) may be considered [115, 116]. Prior to surgical intervention, a comprehensive immunological and allergic evaluation must be completed.

14. Patient follow-up and education

Following the initiation of treatment, patients should be monitored at regular intervals for symptom control and quality-of-life improvement.

14.1 Clinical follow-up parameters

- Symptom assessment: TNSS (Total Nasal Symptom Score), VAS (Visual Analog Scale) [117, 118]
- Quality of Life: RQLQ (Rhinoconjunctivitis Quality of Life Questionnaire) [119]
- Adverse effects of medication and treatment adherence
- For patients receiving AIT: CSMS (Combined Symptom and Medication Score) [120].

14.2 Frequency of follow-up

TNSS and VAS are commonly used as follow-up parameters [121]. During the first month, evaluations every 2–4 weeks are recommended. For stable patients, monitoring every 3–6 months is sufficient. Patients undergoing AIT should be evaluated annually.

14.3 Patient education and counseling

Patients should be informed about the underlying cause of the disease, potential triggers, and preventive strategies. Instructions on the correct use of medications (particularly proper intranasal spray technique), the process of immunotherapy, the expected improvement timeline, and the importance of patience and adherence should be clearly explained.

15. Conclusion and future perspectives

AR is a common disease affecting millions worldwide, with a significant negative impact on quality of life and a substantial economic burden on healthcare systems. Its pathophysiology is shaped by the interaction of genetic predisposition, environmental factors, and IgE-mediated immune responses. Although symptoms are often characteristic, AR may overlap with other types of rhinitis, complicating the diagnostic process. Currently, diagnosis can be established with relative ease through detailed evaluation of clinical symptoms, physical examination findings, and objective tests demonstrating sensitization. The most critical factor in diagnosis is establishing a clear clinical correlation between patient symptoms and allergen sensitization. Management requires a multidisciplinary approach. Pharmacological agents, particularly INCS and antihistamines, are effective and safe for symptom control. Supportive measures, such as allergen avoidance and nasal saline irrigation, also contribute to therapy. AIT remains the only treatment capable of providing both symptomatic relief and long-term disease-modifying effects. With proper patient selection and consistent application, it holds the potential to alter the natural course of the disease.

In the future, more personalized treatment strategies will come to the forefront in AR management. The widespread use of molecular allergy diagnostics will facilitate precise allergen component selection in immunotherapy. Moreover, biologic agents that modulate the immune response (e.g. anti-IgE, anti-IL-4Rα, anti-TSLP) offer promising therapeutic options, particularly for patients with polysensitization or resistance to conventional therapies. In conclusion, successful AR management requires consideration of the disease's heterogeneous nature, environmental influences, and individual variability. Earlydiagnosis, appropriate therapy, and regular follow-up not only improve patient quality of life but may also prevent the development of comorbidities such as asthma.

Author details

Kubra Yırgın and Mehmet Halil Celiksoy*
University of Health Sciences, Basaksehir Cam and Sakura City Hospital, Department of Pediatric Allergy and Immunology, Istanbul, Turkey

*Address all correspondence to: mhceliksoy@gmail.com

References

[1] Wise SK, Damask C, Roland LT, et al. International consensus statement on allergy and rhinology: Allergic rhinitis – 2023. International Forum of Allergy & Rhinology. 2023;**13**:293–859

[2] Giavina-Bianchi P, Aun MV, Takejima P, et al. United airway disease: Current perspectives. Journal of Asthma and Allergy. 2016;**9**:93–100

[3] Akdis CA. 2021. Does the epithelial barrier hypothesis explain the increase in allergy, autoimmunity and other chronic conditions? Nature Reviews Immunology. **21**(11):739–751. DOI: 10.1038/s41577-021-00538-7

[4] Asher MI, Montefort S, Björkstén B, Lai CK, Strachan DP, Weiland SK, Williams H; ISAAC Phase Three Study Group. Worldwide time trends in the prevalence of symptoms of asthma, allergic rhinoconjunctivitis, and eczema in childhood: ISAAC Phases One and Three repeat multicountry cross-sectional surveys. The Lancet. 2006;**368**(9537):733–743. DOI: 10.1016/S0140-6736(06)69283-0

[5] Bousquet J, Khaltaev N, Cruz AA, et al. Allergic Rhinitis and its impact on Asthma (ARIA) 2008 update (in collaboration with the World Health Organization, GA(2)LEN and AllerGen). Allergy. 2008;**63**(86):8–160. DOI: 10.1111/j.1398-9995.2007.01620.x

[6] Pawankar R, G.w C, S.t H, et al. The WAO White Book on Allergy, 2013. Available from: WAO-WhiteBook-2013.pdf. [Accessed: 2025-August-17]

[7] Dykewicz MS, Wallace DV, Amrol DJ, et al. Rhinitis 2020: A practice parameter update. The Journal of Allergy and Clinical Immunology. 2020;**146**(4):721–767. DOI: 10.1016/j.jaci.2020.07.007

[8] Brozek JL, Bousquet J, Baena-Cagnani CE, et al. Allergic Rhinitis and its Impact on Asthma (ARIA) guidelines: 2010 revision. Journal of Allergy and Clinical Immunology. 2010;**126**(3):466–476. DOI: 10.1016/j.jaci.2010.06.047

[9] Nur Husna SM, Tan HT, Md Shukri N, et al. Allergic Rhinitis: A clinical and pathophysiological overview. Frontiers in Medicine Lausanne. 2022;**9**:874114. DOI: 10.3389/fmed.2022.874114

[10] Liva GA, Karatzanis AD, Prokopakis EP. 2021. Review of Rhinitis: Classification, types, pathophysiology. Journal of Clinical Medicine. **10**(14):3183. DOI: 10.3390/jcm10143183

[11] Aït-Khaled N, Pearce N, Anderson HR, et al. Global map of the prevalence of symptoms of rhinoconjunctivitis in children: The international study of Asthma and allergies in childhood (ISAAC) Phase Three. Allergy. 2009;**64**(1):123–148. DOI: 10.1111/j.1398-9995.2008.01884.x

[12] Licari A, Magri P, De Silvestri A, et al. Epidemiology of Allergic Rhinitis in children: A systematic review and meta-analysis. The Journal of Allergy and Clinical Immunology in Practice. 2023;**11**(8):2547–2556. DOI: 10.1016/j.jaip.2023.05.016

[13] Cheng M, Dai Q, Liu Z, et al. New progress in pediatric allergic rhinitis. Frontiers in Immunology. 2024;**15**:1452410. DOI: 10.3389/fimmu.2024.1452410

[14] Xing Y, Wong GW. 2022. Environmental Influences and Allergic Diseases in the Asia-Pacific Region: What will happen in next 30 years? Allergy, Asthma & Immunology Research. **14**(1):21–39. DOI: 10.4168/aair.2022.14.1.21

[15] Haahtela T, Holgate S, Pawankar R, et al. The biodiversity hypothesis and allergic disease: World allergy organization position statement. World Allergy Organization Journal. 2013;**6**(1):3. DOI: 10.1186/1939-4551-6-3

[16] Falcon RMG, Caoili SEC. Immunologic, genetic, and ecological interplay of factors involved in allergic diseases. Frontiers in Allergy. 2023; **4**. 1215616. DOI: 10.3389/falgy.2023.1215616

[17] Özdemir Ö. 2016. Variable prevalence of allergic rhinitis and risk factors affecting the prevalence. The Turkish Journal of Ear Nose and Throat. **26**(6):371–382. DOI: 10.5606/kbbihtisas.2016.97059

[18] Wang J, Zhou Y, Zhang H, et al. Pathogenesis of allergic diseases and implications for therapeutic interventions. Signal Transduction and Targeted Therapy. 2023;**8**(1):138. DOI: 10.1038/s41392-023-01344-4

[19] Chen R, An W, Liu X, et al. Risk factors of allergic rhinitis and its prevention strategies. Frontiers in Allergy. 2024;**5**:1509552. DOI: 10.3389/falgy.2024.1509552

[20] Choi BY, Han M, Kwak JW, et al. Genetics and epigenetics in Allergic Rhinitis. Genes (Basel). 2021;**12**(12):2004. DOI: 10.3390/genes12122004

[21] Bousquet J, Anto JM, Bachert C, et al. Allergic rhinitis. Nature Reviews Disease Primers. 2020;**6**(1):95. DOI: 10.1038/s41572-020-00227-0

[22] Ogulur I, Mitamura Y, Yazici D, et al. Type 2 immunity in allergic diseases. Cellular and Molecular Immunology. 2025;**22**(3):211–242. DOI: 10.1038/s41423-025-01261-2

[23] Castillo EF, Zheng H, Yang XO. Orchestration of epithelial-derived cytokines and innate immune cells in allergic airway inflammation. Cytokine & Growth Factor Reviews. 2018;**39**:19–25. DOI: 10.1016/j.cytogfr.2017.11.004

[24] Lu HF, Zhou YC, Yang LT, et al. Involvement and repair of epithelial barrier dysfunction in allergic diseases. Frontiers in Immunology. 2024;**15**:1348272. DOI: 10.3389/fimmu.2024.1348272

[25] Goleva E, Berdyshev E, Leung DY. 2019. Epithelial barrier repair and prevention of allergy. Journal of Clinical Investigation. **129**(4):1463–1474. DOI: 10.1172/JCI124608

[26] Gu S, Wang R, Zhang W, et al. The production, function, and clinical applications of IL-33 in type 2 inflammation-related respiratory diseases. Frontiers in Immunology. 2024;**15**:1436437. DOI: 10.3389/fimmu.2024.1436437

[27] Duchesne M, Okoye I, Lacy P. Epithelial cell alarmin cytokines: Frontline mediators of the asthma inflammatory response. Frontiers in Immunology. 2022; **13**. 975914. DOI: 10.3389/fimmu.2022.975914

[28] Stefanovic N, Irvine AD. 2024. Filaggrin and beyond: New insights into the skin barrier in atopic dermatitis and allergic diseases, from genetics to

therapeutic perspectives. Annals of Allergy Asthma & Immunology. **132** (2):187–195. DOI: 10.1016/j.anai.2023.09.009

[29] McCoy KD, Ignacio A, Geuking MB. Microbiota and type 2 immune responses. Current Opinion in Immunology. 2018;**54**:20–27. DOI: 10.1016/j.coi.2018.05.009

[30] Gauvreau GM, Bergeron C, Boulet LP, et al. Sounding the alarmins-The role of alarmin cytokines in asthma. Allergy. 2023;**78**(2):402–417. DOI: 10.1111/all.15609

[31] Papadopoulos NG, Bernstein JA, Demoly P, et al. Phenotypes and endotypes of rhinitis and their impact on management: A PRACTALL report. Allergy. 2015;**70**(5):474–494. DOI: 10.1111/all.12573

[32] Bousquet J, Van Cauwenberge P, Khaltaev N; Aria Workshop Group; World Health Organization. Allergic rhinitis and its impact on asthma. The Journal of Allergy and Clinical Immunology. 2001;**108**(5 Suppl): S147–S334. DOI: 10.1067/mai.2001.118891

[33] Cingi C, Catli T. 2012. Phenotyping of allergic rhinitis. Current Allergy and Asthma Reports. **12**(2):115–119. DOI: 10.1007/s11882-012-0243-x

[34] Deb A, Mukherjee S, Saha BK, et al. Profile of patients with Allergic Rhinitis (AR): A clinic based cross-sectional study from Kolkata, India. Journal of Clinical and Diagnostic Research : JCDR. 2014;**8**(1):67–70. DOI: 10.7860/JCDR/2014/6812.3958

[35] Terada T, Kawata R. 2022. Diagnosis and treatment of local Allergic Rhinitis. Pathogens. **11** (1):80. DOI: 10.3390/pathogens11010080

[36] Özdemir O. 2018. Local Allergic Rhinitis (Entopy): Review of the literature. Istanbul Medical Journal. **19** (3):194–201. DOI: 10.5152/imj.2018.66563

[37] Scadding GK, Kariyawasam HH, Scadding G, et al. BSACI guideline for the diagnosis and management of allergic and non-allergic rhinitis (Revised Edition 2017; First edition 2007). Clinical and Experimental Allergy. 2017;**47**(7):856–889. DOI: 10.1111/cea.12953

[38] Hellings PW, Klimek L, Cingi C, et al. Non-allergic rhinitis: Position paper of the European Academy of Allergy and Clinical Immunology. Allergy. 2017;**72**(11):1657–1665. DOI: 10.1111/all.13200

[39] Agache I, Akdis CA. 2019. Precision medicine and phenotypes, endotypes, genotypes, regiotypes, and theratypes of allergic diseases. Journal of Clinical Investigation. **129**(4):1493–1503. DOI: 10.1172/JCI124611

[40] Wallace DV, Dykewicz MS, Bernstein DI, et al. The diagnosis and management of rhinitis: An updated practice parameter. Journal of Allergy and Clinical Immunology. 2008;**122**(2 Suppl):S1–S84. DOI: 10.1016/j.jaci.2008.06.003

[41] Nathan RA. 2007. The burden of allergic rhinitis. Allergy and Asthma Proceedings. **28**(1):3–9. DOI: 10.2500/aap.2007.28.2934

[42] Craig TJ, McCann JL, Gurevich F, et al. The correlation between allergic rhinitis and sleep disturbance. Journal of Allergy and Clinical Immunology.

2004;**114**(5 Suppl):S139–S145. DOI: 10.1016/j.jaci.2004.08.044

[43] Smolensky MH, Reinberg A, Labrecque G. 1995. Twenty-four hour pattern in symptom intensity of viral and allergic rhinitis: Treatment implications. Journal of Allergy and Clinical Immunology. **95**(5):1084–1096. DOI: 10.1016/s0091-6749(95)70212-1

[44] Shedden A. 2005. Impact of nasal congestion on quality of life and work productivity in allergic rhinitis: Findings from a large online survey. Treatments in Respiratory Medicine. **4**(6):439–446. DOI: 10.2165/00151829-200504060-00007

[45] Narasimhan G, Deshmukh PT, Gaurkar SS, et al. A comprehensive review exploring Allergic Rhinitis with Nasal Polyps: Mechanisms, management, and emerging therapies. Cureus. 2024;**16**(4):e59191. DOI: 10.7759/cureus.59191

[46] Stuck BA, Hummel T. 2015. Olfaction in allergic rhinitis: A systematic review. Journal of Allergy and Clinical Immunology. **136**(6): 1460–1470. DOI: 10.1016/j.jaci.2015.08.003

[47] Scadding GK, Smith PK, Blaiss M, et al. Allergic Rhinitis in childhood and the new EUFOREA algorithm. Frontiers in Allergy. 2021;**2**:706589. DOI: 10.3389/falgy.2021.706589

[48] Rotiroti G, Roberts G, Scadding GK. 2015. Rhinitis in children: Common clinical presentations and differential diagnoses. Pediatric Allergy and Immunology. **26**(2):103–110. DOI: 10.1111/pai.12339

[49] Chen Y, Lin L, Hong B, et al. Association of allergic symptoms in the first 2 years of life with sleep outcomes among Chinese toddlers. Frontiers in Pediatrics. 2022;**9**:791369. DOI: 10.3389/fped.2021.791369

[50] Ma Y, Tang J, Wen Y, et al. Associations of sleep problems with asthma and allergic rhinitis among Chinese preschoolers. Scientific Reports. 2022;**12**(1):8102. DOI: 10.1038/s41598-022-12207-3

[51] Chang HY, Seo JH, Kim HY, et al. Allergic diseases in preschoolers are associated with psychological and behavioural problems. Allergy, Asthma & Immunology Research. 2013;**5**(5):315–321. DOI: 10.4168/aair.2013.5.5.315

[52] Gelardi M, Giancaspro R, Boni E, et al. Rhinitis in the geriatric population: Epidemiological and cytological aspects. Geriatrics (Basel). 2025;**10**(2):50. DOI: 10.3390/geriatrics10020050

[53] Kotz S, Pechtold L, Jörres RA, Nowak D, Chaker AM. Occupational rhinitis. Allergologie Select. 2021;**5**: 51–56. DOI: 10.5414/ALX02165E

[54] Çakan D, Öztürk E. 2022. The effects of Allergic Rhinitis on sleep quality. Journal of Academic Research in Medicine. **12**(1):5–9. DOI: 10.4274/jarem.galenos.2021.28199

[55] Almalki ZA, Atalla AA, Altalhi FM, et al. The prevalence and impact of Allergic Rhinitis on academic performance and quality of life among medical students in Saudi Arabia. Cureus. 2023;**15**(7):e42342. DOI: 10.7759/cureus.42342

[56] Kimchi N, Bielory L. 2020. The allergic eye: Recommendations about pharmacotherapy and recent therapeutic agents. Current Opinion in

Allergy & Clinical Immunology. **20** (4):414–420. DOI: 10.1097/ ACI.0000000000000669

[57] Mehta R. Allergy and Asthma: Allergic Rhinitis and Allergic Conjunctivitis. FP Essentials. 2018;**472**:11–15

[58] Spector SL. 1997. Overview of comorbid associations of allergic rhinitis. Journal of Allergy and Clinical Immunology. **99**(2):S773–S780. DOI: 10.1016/s0091-6749(97)70126-x

[59] Laidlaw TM, Mullol J, Woessner KM, Amin N, Mannent LP. 2021. Chronic Rhinosinusitis with Nasal Polyps and Asthma. The Journal of Allergy and Clinical Immunology in Practice. **9**(3):1133–1141. DOI: 10.1016/ j.jaip.2020.09.063

[60] Cao Y, Wu S, Zhang L, Yang Y, Cao S, Li Q. Association of allergic rhinitis with obstructive sleep apnea: A meta-analysis. Medicine (Baltimore). 2018; **97**(51):e13783. DOI: 10.1097/ MD.0000000000013783

[61] Knudgaard MH, Andreasen TH, Ravnborg N, et al. Rhinitis prevalence and association with atopic dermatitis: A systematic review and meta-analysis. Annals of Allergy Asthma & Immunology. 2021;**127** (1):49–56.e1. DOI: 10.1016/j.anai. 2021.02.026

[62] Kung YM, Tsai PY, Chang YH, et al. Allergic rhinitis is a risk factor of gastro-esophageal reflux disease regardless of the presence of asthma. Scientific Reports. 2019;**9**(1): 15535. DOI: 10.1038/s41598-019- 51661-4

[63] Yang L, Fu J, Zhou Y. Research progress in atopic march. Frontiers in Immunology. 2020;**11**:1907. DOI: 10.33 89/fimmu.2020.01907

[64] Bantz SK, Zhu Z, Zheng T. 2014. The atopic march: progression from atopic dermatitis to Allergic Rhinitis and asthma. Journal of Clinical & Cellular Immunology. **5**(2):202. DOI: 10.4172/2155-9899.1000202

[65] Paller AS, Spergel JM, Mina-Osorio P, Irvine AD. 2019. The atopic march and atopic multimorbidity: Many trajectories, many pathways. Journal of Allergy and Clinical Immunology. **143** (1):46–55. DOI: 10.1016/j.jaci.2018. 11.006

[66] Weaver-Agostoni J, Kosak Z, Bartlett S.Allergic Rhinitis: Rapid evidence review. . American Family Physician. 2023;**107**(5):466–473

[67] Ansotegui IJ, Melioli G, Canonica GW, et al. IgE allergy diagnostics and other relevant tests in allergy, a World Allergy Organization position paper. World Allergy Organization Journal. 2020;**13**(2):100080. DOI: 10.1016/j. waojou.2019.100080

[68] Testera-Montes A, Jurado R, Salas M, Eguiluz-Gracia I, Mayorga C. Diagnostic Tools in Allergic Rhinitis. Frontiers in Allergy. 2021; **2**. 721851. DOI: 10.3389/falgy.2021.721851

[69] Caruso C, Giancaspro R, Guida G, et al. Nasal cytology: A easy diagnostic tool in precision medicine for inflammation in epithelial barrier damage in the nose. A perspective mini review. Frontiers in Allergy. 2022;**3**:768408. DOI: 10.3389/ falgy.2022.768408

[70] Myszkowska D, Bazgier M, Brońska S, et al. Scraping nasal cytology in the diagnostics of rhinitis and the

comorbidities. Scientific Reports. 2022;**12**(1):14492. DOI: 10.1038/s41598-022-18734-3

[71] Cho SH, Nanda A, Keswani A, et al. Nasal allergen challenge (NAC): Practical aspects and applications from an EU/US perspective-a work group report of the AAAAI Rhinitis. Rhinosinusitis and Ocular Allergy Committee. Journal of Allergy and Clinical Immunology. 2023;**151**(5): 1215–1222.e4. DOI: 10.1016/j.jaci.2023.02.014

[72] Uzzaman A, Metcalfe DD, Komarow HD. 2006. Acoustic rhinometry in the practice of allergy. Annals of Allergy Asthma & Immunology. **97**(6):745–799. DOI: 10.1016/S1081-1206(10)60964-7

[73] Jareoncharsri P, Thitadilok V, Bunnag C, Ungkanont K, Voraprayoon S, Tansuriyawong P.Nasal endoscopic findings in patients with perennial allergic rhinitis. Asian Pacific Journal of Allergy & Immunology. 1999;**17**(4):261–267

[74] Sara KB, Rupa V, Jeyaseelan L. 2022. Changes in olfaction & quality of life following standard medical therapy in patients with intermittent & persistent allergic rhinitis. Indian Journal of Medical Research. **155** (3&4):373–379. DOI: 10.4103/ijmr.IJMR_1517_19

[75] Sur DKC, Plesa ML.Chronic Nonallergic Rhinitis. American Family Physician. 2018;**98**(3):171–176

[76] Cho SH, Ledford D, Lockey RF. 2020. Medical Management Strategies in Acute and Chronic Rhinosinusitis. The Journal of Allergy and Clinical Immunology in Practice. **8**(5): 1559–1564. DOI: 10.1016/j.jaip.2020.02.020

[77] Quillen DM, Feller DB.Diagnosing rhinitis: Allergic vs. nonallergic. . American Family Physician. 2006;**73** (9):1583–1590

[78] Tomé M, Lourenço O. 2023. Avoidance Measures for Patients with Allergic Rhinitis: A Scoping Review. Children (Basel, Switzerland). **10** (2):300. DOI: 10.3390/children10020300

[79] Wang Y, Jin L, Liu SX, et al. Role of nasal saline irrigation in the treatment of allergic rhinitis in children and adults: A systematic analysis. Allergologia Et Immunopathologia. 2020;**48**(4): 360–367. DOI: 10.1016/j.aller.2020.01.002

[80] Head K, Snidvongs K, Glew S, et al. Saline irrigation for allergic rhinitis. The Cochrane Database of Systematic Reviews. 2018;**6**(6):CD012597. DOI: 10.1002/14651858.CD012597.pub2

[81] Soe KK, Krikeerati T, Pheerapanyawaranun C, et al. Comparative efficacy and acceptability of licensed dose intranasal corticosteroids for moderate-to-severe allergic rhinitis: A systematic review and network meta-analysis. Frontiers in Pharmacology. 2023;**14**:1184552. DOI: 10.3389/fphar.2023.1184552

[82] Daley-Yates PT, Larenas-Linnemann D, Bhargave C, et al. Intranasal corticosteroids: Topical potency, systemic activity and therapeutic index. Journal of Asthma and Allergy. 2021;**14**: 1093–1104

[83] Linton S, Hossenbaccus L, Ellis AK. 2023. Evidence-based use of antihistamines for treatment of allergic conditions. Annals of Allergy

Asthma & Immunology. **131**(4):412–420. DOI: 10.1016/j.anai.2023.07.019

[84] JA B, JS B, Makol R, et al. Allergic Rhinitis: A review. JAMA. 2024;**331**(10):866–877. DOI: 10.1001/jama.2024.0530

[85] Bousquet J, Klimek L, Kuhl HC, et al. A double-blind, placebo-controlled trial of the efficacy and safety of two doses of azelastine hydrochloride in perennial allergic rhinitis. Frontiers in Allergy. 2023;**4**:1244012. DOI: 10.3389/falgy.2023.1244012

[86] Tunca S, Yilmaz O, Ocalan M, Arga M, Cavkaytar O, Ozceker D, Kiliç M, Duksal F, Can D, Sancakli O, Mş K, Ercan N, Gunaydin NC, Aydogan M, Demir E, Sancak R, Sik K, Sapan N, Demir AU, Bilac O, Misirlioglu ED, Turkeli A, Artac H, Gungor HE, Cokugras H, Orhan F, Bingol A, Uysal P, Keles S, Ozhan AK, Tuncel T, Keskin O, Arik E, Ö Ö, Can C, Altinel N, Harmanci K, Simsek Y, Altintas DU, Ozmen S, Uzuner N, Canıtez Y, Yüksel H. Potentially overlooked risk for neuropsychiatric symptoms in children: Montelukast treatment. Journal of Paediatrics and Child Health. 2025. doi:10.1111/jpc.70092

[87] Hox V, Lourijsen E, Jordens A, et al. Benefits and harm of systemic steroids for short- and long-term use in rhinitis and rhinosinusitis: An EAACI position paper. Clinical & Translational Allergy. 2020;**10**:1

[88] Ratner PH, Ehrlich PM, Fineman SM, Meltzer EO, Skoner DP. 2002. Use of intranasal cromolyn sodium for allergic rhinitis. Mayo Clinic Proceedings. **77**(4):350–354. DOI: 10.4065/77.4.350

[89] Sobczak M, Kowal K, Pawliczak R. 2025. Are there effective methods to reduce exposure to house dust mite allergens? A meta-analysis of randomized clinical trials. International Forum of Allergy & Rhinology. **15**(8):792–802. DOI: 10.1002/alr.23565

[90] Terreehorst I, Hak E, Oosting AJ, et al. Evaluation of impermeable covers for bedding in patients with allergic rhinitis. New England Journal of Medicine. 2003;**349**(3):237–246. DOI: 10.1056/NEJMoa023171

[91] Klain A, Senatore AA, Licari A, et al. The prevention of house dust mite allergies in pediatric asthma. Children (Basel, Switzerland). 2024;**11**(4):469. DOI: 10.3390/children11040469

[92] Bergmann KC, Berger M, Klimek L, et al. Nonpharmacological measures to prevent allergic symptoms in pollen allergy: A critical review. Allergologie Select. 2021;**5**:349–360

[93] WHO Guidelines for Indoor Air Quality: Dampness and Mould. Geneva: World Health Organization; 2009. Available from: https://www.ncbi.nlm.nih.gov/books/NBK143941/ [Accessed: 2025-August-17]

[94] Jaakkola MS, Quansah R, Hugg TT, Heikkinen SA, Jaakkola JJ. 2013. Association of indoor dampness and molds with rhinitis risk: A systematic review and meta-analysis. Journal of Allergy and Clinical Immunology. **132**(5):1099–1110.e18. DOI: 10.1016/j.jaci.2013.07.028

[95] Kilburn S, Lasserson TJ, McKean M. Pet allergen control measures for allergic asthma in children and adults. The Cochrane Database of Systematic Reviews. 2003; **2001**(1):CD002989. DOI: 10.1002/14651858.CD002989

[96] An W, Li T, Tian X, et al. Allergies to allergens from cats and dogs: A review and update on sources, pathogenesis, and Strategies. International Journal of Molecular Sciences. 2024;**25**(19):10520. DOI: 10.3390/ijms251910520

[97] Portnoy J, Chew GL, Phipatanakul W, et al. Environmental assessment and exposure reduction of cockroaches: A practice parameter. Journal of Allergy and Clinical Immunology. 2013;**132**(4):802-8.e25. DOI: 10.1016/j.jaci.2013.04.061

[98] Krieger J, Jacobs DE, Ashley PJ, et al. Housing interventions and control of asthma-related indoor biologic agents: A review of the evidence. Journal of Public Health Management and Practice. 2010;**16**(5 Suppl):S11–S20. DOI: 10.1097/PHH.0b013e3181ddcbd9

[99] Chen J, Liu X, Su W, et al. Unveiling the hidden risk: Paternal smoking and alcohol exposure prior to conception as independent factors for allergic rhinitis in children. Frontiers in Pediatrics. 2024;**12**:1394400. DOI: 10.3389/fped.2024.1394400

[100] Yao TC, SW C, Wc C, et al. Exposure to tobacco smoke and childhood rhinitis: A population-based study. Scientific Reports. 2017;**7**:42836. DOI: 10.1038/srep42836

[101] Saulyte J, Regueira C, Montes-Martínez A, Khudyakov P, Takkouche B. Active or passive exposure to tobacco smoking and allergic rhinitis, allergic dermatitis, and food allergy in adults and children: A systematic review and meta-analysis. PLoS Medicine. 2014; **11**(3):e1001611. DOI: 10.1371/journal.pmed.1001611

[102] Alvaro-Lozano M, CA A, Akdis M, et al. EAACI allergen immunotherapy user's guide. Pediatric Allergy and Immunology. 2020;**31**(Suppl 25):1–101. DOI: 10.1111/pai.13189

[103] Roberts G, Pfaar O, Akdis CA, et al. EAACI guidelines on allergen immunotherapy: Allergic rhinoconjunctivitis. Allergy. 2018;**73**(4):765–798. DOI: 10.1111/all.13317

[104] Aboshady OA, Elghanam KM. 2014. Sublingual immunotherapy in allergic rhinitis: Efficacy, safety, adherence and guidelines. Clinical and Experimental Otorhinolaryngology. **7**(4):241–249. DOI: 10.3342/ceo.2014.7.4.241

[105] Dhami S, Nurmatov U, Arasi S, et al. Allergen immunotherapy for allergic rhinoconjunctivitis: A systematic review and meta-analysis. Allergy. 2017;**72**(11):1597–1631. DOI: 10.1111/all.13201

[106] Kim JM, Lin SY, Suarez-Cuervo C, et al. Allergen-specific immunotherapy for pediatric asthma and rhinoconjunctivitis: A systematic review. Pediatrics. 2013;**131**(6):1155–1167. DOI: 10.1542/peds.2013-0343

[107] Giannetti A, Ricci G, Procaccianti M, Santoro A, Safety CC. Efficacy, and preventive role of subcutaneous and sublingual allergen immunotherapy for the treatment of pediatric asthma. Journal of Asthma and Allergy. 2020;**13**:575–587. DOI: 10.2147/JAA.S234280

[108] Wilson DR, Lima MT, Durham SR. 2005. Sublingual immunotherapy for allergic rhinitis: Systematic review

and meta-analysis. Allergy. **60**(1): 4–12. DOI: 10.1111/j.1398-9995.2005. 00699.x

[109] Aissa S, Ben Jazia R, Ayachi J, et al. Critical appraisal of the clinical utility of sublingual immunotherapy in allergy. Contemporary Clinical Trials Communications. 2016;**4**:1–8

[110] Lindqvist M, Leth-Møller KB, Linneberg A, et al. Natural course of pollen-induced allergic rhinitis from childhood to adulthood: A 20-year follow up. Allergy. 2024;**79**(4): 884–893. DOI: 10.1111/all.15927

[111] Acevedo-Prado A, Seoane-Pillado T, López-Silvarrey-Varela A, et al. Association of rhinitis with asthma prevalence and severity. Scientific Reports. 2022;**12**(1):6389. DOI: 10.1038/ s41598-022-10448-w

[112] Tohidinik HR, Mallah N, Takkouche B. History of allergic rhinitis and risk of asthma; a systematic review and meta-analysis. World Allergy Organization Journal. 2019; **12** (10):100069. DOI: 10.1016/j. waojou.2019.100069

[113] Arshad H, Lack G, Durham SR, Penagos M, Larenas-Linnemann D, Halken S. 2024. Prevention is better than cure: Impact of allergen immunotherapy on the progression of airway disease. The Journal of Allergy and Clinical Immunology in Practice. **12**(1):45–56. DOI: 10.1016/j.jaip.2023.10.013

[114] Penagos M, Durham SR. 2022. Allergen immunotherapy for long-term tolerance and prevention. Journal of Allergy and Clinical Immunology. **149** (3):802–811. DOI: 10.1016/j. jaci.2022.01.007

[115] Soumya S, Adegboyega G, Elhassan H. 2021. Surgical approaches for allergic rhinitis: A systematic review protocol. International Journal of Surgery Protocols. **25**(1):178–183. DOI: 10.29337/ijsp.160

[116] Nagalingeswaran A, Kumar RD. 2020. Newer surgical options for nasal allergy. Indian Journal of Otolaryngology and Head & Neck Surgery. **72**(1):133–139. DOI: 10.1007/s 12070-019-01772-1

[117] Florack J, Brighetti MA, Perna S, et al. Comparison of six disease severity scores for allergic rhinitis against pollen counts a prospective analysis at population and individual level. Pediatric Allergy and Immunology. 2016;**27**(4):382–390. DOI: 10.1111/ pai.12562

[118] Klimek L, Bergmann KC, Biedermann T, et al. Visual analogue scales (VAS): Measuring instruments for the documentation of symptoms and therapy monitoring in cases of allergic rhinitis in everyday health care: Position paper of the german society of allergology (AeDA) and the german society of allergy and clinical immunology (DGAKI), ENT section, in collaboration with the working group on clinical Immunology, Allergology and environmental medicine of the german society of otorhinolaryngology, Head and neck surgery (DGHNOKHC). Allergo Journal International. 2017;**26** (1):16–24. DOI: 10.1007/s40629-016-0 006-7

[119] Juniper EF, Guyatt GH. 1991. Development and testing of a new measure of health status for clinical trials in rhinoconjunctivitis. Clinical and Experimental Allergy. **21**

(1):77–83. DOI: 10.1111/j.1365-2222.1991.tb00807.x

[120] Sousa-Pinto B, Azevedo LF, Jutel M, et al. Development and validation of combined symptom-medication scores for allergic rhinitis. Allergy. 2022;**77**(7):2147–2162. DOI: 10.1111/all.15199

[121] Zhang K, Li AR, Miglani A, Nguyen SA, Schlosser RJ. 2022. Effect of medical therapy in allergic rhinitis: A systematic review and meta-analysis. American Journal of Rhinology & Allergy. **36**(2):269–280. DOI: 10.1177/19458924211041438